Praise for *Allergy Guide*
Comments from Andrew Weil, MD

"The conventional management of allergic conditions relies on suppressive drugs that often lose effectiveness over time. In this book, Dr. Elizabeth Smoots does a terrific job of explaining how to use an integrative approach that can actually help the immune system unlearn allergic reactivity. She stresses the usefulness of dietary change, natural remedies, and mind-body therapies along with the pros and cons of the standard drugs. Essential reading for anyone who suffers from allergy."

Andrew Weil, MD
Author of *Spontaneous Healing* and *Natural Health, Natural Medicine*
Director, Arizona Center for Integrative Medicine
Clinical Professor of Medicine
Jones-Lovell Endowed Chair in Integrative Rheumatology
University of Arizona College of Medicine
Tucson, Arizona

ALLERGY
GUIDE

Elizabeth Smoots, MD

ALLERGY

GUIDE

Alternative & Conventional Solutions

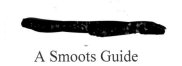

A Smoots Guide

ISBN-13: 978-1483957418 (paperback)
ISBN-10: 1483957411 (paperback)
ISBN-13: 978-1626753853 (e-book)

Cover images of allergy treatments: An aromatherapy diffuser and a cup of herbal tea

Dedication

৪০৫

To those committed to bringing
prevention and wellness back into health care

Disclaimer

ℰꙅ⳩

This book provides general health information intended for educational purposes only. It does not replace personalized care and treatment by a licensed medical professional. Health care must be individualized since a treatment that helps one may be harmful to another. Always consult your health care provider before undertaking any activity or adhering to any information or recommendations in this book. The author makes no guarantees and disclaims all liability in connection with the use in any way or by any means of this book.

Table of Contents

Preface 15

A Whole Person Approach to Self-Healing 17

Part I Allergy Basics 21

Chapter 1 Brief Overview of Allergies.......................... 23

An Epidemic of Allergies 23

Types of Allergic Conditions 24

Allergy-Related Problems 28

Chapter 2 Diagnostic Steps...................................... 31

Risk Factors 31

Diagnostic Tests 32

Part II Conventional Care of Allergic Conditions........... 39

Chapter 3 Self Care... 41

Lifestyle Habits... 41

Home Remedies 45

Health Care Savvy 47

Chapter 4 Avoidance of Triggers............................... 51

Pollens 52

Dust Mites 53

Molds 54

Cockroaches 55

Dander from Pets 55

Chemicals & Irritants 56

Foods 58

Chapter 5 Over-the-Counter Medications...................61

Saline Sprays...61

Antihistamines 62

Decongestants 64

Mast Cell Stabilizers.....................................65

Chapter 6 Prescription Medications 67

Antihistamines 69

Mast Cell Stabilizers.....................................70

Anticholinergic Agents 71

Corticosteroids 72

Epinephrine 74

Beta Agonists...75

Leukotriene Modifiers...................................76

Antibody Neutralizers...................................77

Chapter 7 Immunotherapy 79

Allergy Shots..80

Emerging Treatments 81

Part III Alternative Therapies for Allergic Conditions....83

Chapter 8 Nutrition 85

Dietary Protein.. 85

Dairy Products...86

Healthy & Unhealthy Fats............................. 87

Anti-inflammatory Diet 90

Low-Glycemic Diet.......................................95

Food Allergies & Sensitivities 96

Chapter 9 Aromatherapy & Essential Oils.................. 97

    Inhalation of Essential Oils....................... 98

    Topical Use of Essential Oils 101

Chapter 10 Herbal Remedies 105

    Herbs for Allergy Relief........................... 106

    Herbs to Aid Respiratory Tract................... 110

    Herbs for Immune Support 113

Chapter 11 Dietary Supplements.................... 117

    Principal Supplements 118

    Other Supplements 121

Chapter 12 Mind-Body Therapies 125

    Journaling 126

    Breathwork 127

    Progressive Muscle Relaxation 128

    Guided Imagery................................... 129

    Meditation 130

    Hypnotherapy 131

    Biofeedback 132

Chapter 13 Manual Medicine 135

    Osteopathic Treatment........................... 135

    Craniosacral Therapy 136

    Massage Therapy................................. 137

Chapter 14 Whole Medical Systems 139

    Traditional Chinese Medicine 139

    Ayurveda.. 141

Homeopathy...142

Part IV Prevention of Allergic Conditions....................147

Chapter 15 Allergy Prevention..............................149

Diet & Lifestyle Changes....................................149

Friendly Intestinal Flora....................................151

Appendices...153

Appendix A Sample Elimination Diet......................155

Appendix B Moved to Exercise..............................159

Appendix C How Much Calcium Are You Getting?..163

Appendix D Calcium Content of Foods...................167

Appendix E The "Dirty Dozen".............................169

Appendix F The "Clean Fifteen"...........................171

Appendix G Glossary of Herbal & Botanical Terms....173

About the Author..175

Sample of Dr. Elizabeth's Blog A Whole Health Life 177

Living a Whole Health Life...................................178

Biography Dr. Elizabeth Smoots...........................181

Preface

৪৩০৪

A Whole Person Approach to Self-Healing

✂☙❡

We have an ailing health care system in this country. A standard medical visit in the U.S. typically results in a drug solution to a single problem. If you have more than one problem, you may well be told to return for help another day. All too often, when your tests come back normal even though you still feel ill, you are told nothing is wrong. You have reached the end of the line for conventional medical care.

Obviously, several serious problems exist with this model. In my roles as an integrative medicine physician, family medicine doctor, health writer, medical editor and patient, I have witnessed the breakdown of a health care system ruled by health insurance companies and large drug corporations. These special interests have come to stand between the physician and patient at the sacrifice of many areas of health.

Health Care Problems

For starters, a growing number of people are not receiving quality care for their health conditions. Our country's disease-driven approach has led to fragmented care that is often ineffective and impersonal. The lack of comprehensive care is especially felt with chronic ailments like diabetes, heart disease, asthma, high blood pressure and depression.

Research definitively shows that most of these conditions can be slowed down or prevented with healthier ways of living. Yet, the U.S. health care system does not adequately support people through the lifestyle changes needed to nip these diseases in the bud.

Instead of embracing healthier lifestyles, we largely turn to drugs. But drugs are not always the best solutions since they don't address the root causes of illness. Medications are also very costly and can have serious side effects. Plus, the greater the number of drugs you take, the higher the risk of dangerous interactions with other drugs, food, herbs and dietary supplements. Sometimes the treatment truly becomes worse than the disease.

Largely ignored within our medical system are a whole host of alternatives: Herbs that are gentle yet effective. Dietary supplements that fill gaps left by an inadequate diet or poor digestion. Whole systems like homeopathy and Chinese medicine that look at the mind, body and spirit of an individual in assessing illness. Mind-body therapies that address mental and emotional states as well as bodily health. Physical exercise and manual medicine techniques that make the connection between our musculoskeletal systems and our internal organs. Energy healing that aims to diagnose and treat imbalances in the subtle energy field surrounding each person.

It is true that surgery and drugs have their place. But we rely on the big guns and magic bullets too much. This country's people use drugs when diet, exercise or a few simple herbs would be safer and more effective. Yet there is another way: We could save stronger and riskier treatments for times when they're truly needed, and start with milder and gentler remedies instead.

Elizabeth Smoots MD

Our penchant for turning to more and more technology and surgical procedures has not led to better health. In fact, the opposite is true. Despite medical expenses that are more than twice as high as other Western nations, the health of U.S. citizens ranks only twelfth out of the top 13 industrialized countries in the world. And our life expectancy compared to citizens in most other nations has fallen to a low of 51st place. This data from the World Health Organization and the U.S. Central Intelligence Agency clearly shows we're slipping behind. So what are we to do?

Health Care Solutions

Many feel that health care must become more prevention-oriented, more patient-centered, and more personalized. My belief in these qualities, which offer real solutions to our problems, led to my becoming an integrative medicine physician. I received specialized training in this field during my fellowship at the world-renowned Arizona Center for Integrative Medicine founded by Andrew Weil, MD, at the University of Arizona College of Medicine. This type of medical care incorporates both conventional and alternative therapies that are backed by scientific research. Preventive therapies like diet, exercise and healthy lifestyle habits form the foundation of integrative medicine. Practitioners emphasize building a partnership with patients to provide better and more comprehensive care for each individual's mind, body and spirit.

The field of integrative medicine embraces evidence-based alternative approaches to treating illness. Examples of popular alternative therapies include herbal remedies, dietary supplements, meditation, breathing exercises, guided imagery, energy healing and hypnosis. Acupuncture, ayurvedic medicine, homeopathy, naturopathy, chiropractic or osteopathic manipulation, and massage therapy are some of the many other alternatives that can be utilized when appropriate. The discipline's basic tenet is to take advantage of natural and less invasive solutions whenever possible.

Integrative medicine also recognizes that conventional therapies such as medications or surgery are the most effective options for treating certain disorders. In the treatment of urgent and acute illness, Western medicine has no equal. Antibiotics, vaccines, surgery with sterile technique and anesthesia—these are huge advances that have brought tremendous progress to the field of medicine.

An Integrative Approach

When you are a patient seeking medical care, wouldn't you like to know all of your options? What if someone would sit down with you to explain the alternative and conventional treatments for your health condition and answer your questions? That is what this book series aims to do. With one of my health guides in your hand (or on your screen), you will be better equipped to care for your condition, or know what questions to ask when you visit your health care provider.

The goal of this first book in the series is to inform you of your main allergy options from the fields of alternative and conventional medicine. Keep in mind that the best treatment mix for you is likely different than for someone else, and finding it often involves a trial and error process. I sincerely hope the whole person approach I'm taking will help you discover effective solutions in your search for wellness.

Elizabeth Smoots, MD
FAAFP, ABFM, Graduate Fellow AZCIM
Author of *Practical Prevention*
Seattle, Washington

Part I
Allergy Basics

ᏧᎳ

Chapter 1
Brief Overview of Allergies

ର୍ଷେ୪୦

Allergies are curious phenomena. They make you react to harmless substances like pollen, dust, mold, food and cat fur that ordinarily don't bother people. These substances cannot hurt us like infectious diseases or animal bites, so your body need not protect against them. Yet it tries to anyway, with potentially harmful signs of disease when you have allergies. What causes this situation to occur?

An Epidemic of Allergies

Certain kinds of allergies have increased dramatically in developed nations over the last century. At present hay fever afflicts one in five people. The frequency of asthma has increased more than 10-fold in the past 40 years. An estimated 60 million people suffer from all types of allergies in the U.S.

While not fully understood, several factors lurk behind the growing allergy epidemic. These include improved sanitation, fewer infections from worms and parasites, greater efficiency of home heating and ventilation, decreased levels of physical activity, and increased consumption of processed foods. Some of these changes have brought progress in terms of fewer deaths from infectious disease. As a whole, however, they have ushered in a higher frequency of hay fever and asthma.

The most popular explanation for the rise in allergies is called the hygiene hypothesis. It argues that better hygiene leads to increased allergic disease. Exposure to germs in early life, the hypothesis goes, influences the normal development and maturation of your immune system. It does this partly by affecting the amounts and types of friendly bacteria living in your intestines. Scientists have discovered the vital role these beneficial bacteria play in regulating your immune system. Not having enough good gut bacteria, or having too many bad ones, can throw your entire body's immunity out of whack. Even a small imbalance can set up a situation that encourages the formation of allergies.

While scientists suspect the growing allergy epidemic starts with reduced germ exposure in childhood, proof of the hygiene hypothesis still remains to be seen. In the meantime, there exists a huge need for more research about the underlying causes of allergies.

Types of Allergic Conditions

Physicians often like to talk about a triad of allergic disease. Hay fever, eczema and asthma are the leading allergic disorders, and all three frequently occur in the same people. The manifestations of allergies are varied, however, and may include the following conditions:

Hay Fever
Allergic rhinitis is the medical term for hay fever. In this condition, your body's response to allergenic substances causes chronic inflammation of the mucous membranes inside your nose. Subsequent exposure to pollens, dust, dander or other allergens can trigger symptoms such as sneezing, itching, nasal congestion, runny nose, post-nasal drip, cough, and tearing eyes. Other signs include fatigue,

irritability, difficulty concentrating, and poor appetite. The condition can occur seasonally or year-round. Many of my patients with allergic rhinitis have perennial symptoms that get worse in the spring, and sometimes in the fall.

Allergic Sinus Problems

If you have allergic rhinitis, you likely have similar inflammatory changes in the linings of your sinuses. Research indicates that the sinus inflammation occurs chronically, just like it does in the nasal passages during hay fever. The medical term for this condition is "allergic rhinosinusitis." Symptoms of the ailment, which may occur upon exposure to allergy-causing substances, include sinus fullness or pressure and post-nasal drip.

Eczema

Also known as atopic dermatitis, the allergic condition consists of itching and inflammation of your skin. Rashes most commonly appear on your hands and feet, front of your arms, and behind your knees. Eczema may also occur on your ankles, wrists, face, neck and upper chest. A viscous cycle of itching and scratching can lead to chronic skin problems such as thickening, cracking or scaling.

Allergic Asthma

Asthma is a chronic inflammatory lung condition in which your airways constrict and dilate and produce extra mucus. The characteristic symptoms consist of coughing, chest tightness, shortness of breath and wheezing. Asthma usually starts and stops in a reversible pattern that waxes and wanes. Considerable variability exists from person to person in the triggers that touch off asthma. Viral infections, cold air, pollutants, physical activity and stress are common inflammatory triggers. Additionally, if you have allergic asthma, you may react to allergy-causing agents such as pollen, animal dander, mold or certain foods.

Eye Allergies

Allergies of the eyes are referred to medically as allergic conjunctivitis. The tell-tale signs of itchy, watery, and red or swollen eyes can occur acutely, seasonally or year-round. Eye allergies can happen alone or be part of the symptom complex of hay fever.

Food Allergies

Allergies to food arise when your body's immune system reacts abnormally to food constituents such as protein. The eight main groups of foods that trigger food allergies are milk, eggs, fish, crustacean shellfish, tree nuts, peanuts, wheat and soybeans. These eight groups account for over 90 percent of food allergies in the U.S., and represent the foods most likely to cause serious reactions.

Symptoms of food allergy usually appear within 24 hours after you eat a food and can range from mild to life threatening. Prolonged effects may last for two to three days, or occasionally longer, after a reaction. The symptoms of food allergy may affect many different areas of your body. A large variety of symptoms are possible.

HEALTH TIP FROM DR. SMOOTS

Food Allergy Symptoms

Ranging from annoying to life threatening, food allergy symptoms can involve almost any part of your body. Examples of symptoms that may occur include:

- Skin: Hives, flushing, eczema, itchy rash, or swelling of the face or extremities
- Eyes: Itching, tearing, redness, or swelling of the skin around the eyes
- Digestive system: Nausea, vomiting, abdominal cramps, diarrhea, blood in the stool
- Nose: Nasal congestion or itching, sneezing, hay fever
- Mouth: Itching, tingling, and swelling of the lips, tongue or mouth
- Throat: Itching or tightness in the throat, hoarseness, hacking cough
- Lungs: Shortness of breath, repeated coughing or wheezing, asthma
- Heart: Weak pulse, low blood pressure, passing out
- Nervous system: Migraine headaches, trouble concentrating or confusion
- Psyche: Anxiety, fatigue, sense of impending doom, or behavior problems such as hyperactivity
- Entire body: Severe reaction with swelling of the tongue and throat, difficulty breathing, loss of consciousness and shock. This condition, called anaphylaxis, is discussed in more detail in the final section of this chapter.

Non-allergic food reactions

Even more common than food allergies are other types of food reactions that are not caused by the immune system. These reactions can cause bothersome symptoms even though they are not true food allergies. Common examples include food intolerances and sensitivities. For instance, people often become lactose intolerant when they are deficient in the enzyme, lactase, needed to digest milk sugar.

Symptoms such as abdominal cramps, gas and bloating develop when they consume greater amounts of dairy products than they can tolerate. Other people develop sensitivities to certain foods or food ingredients such as gluten or fructose. Food additives like monosodium glutamate, sulfites or preservatives are another potential source of sensitivities to food for some people.

Allergy-Related Problems

Allergic conditions are not just a nuisance. Besides being a health threat in their own right, allergies often progress to other allergic conditions. In children with eczema, for instance, nearly 80 percent will go on to develop hay fever or asthma. Up to half of people who have hay fever may eventually suffer from some form of asthma. Studies also show that about three-quarters of people with asthma have associated nasal allergies.

Exactly how are allergies and asthma connected? Recent studies have demonstrated cross talk between the upper and lower airways of the respiratory tract. When a person with hay fever but no asthma is exposed to ragweed or house dust, inflammation flares up not only in the nose but also in the lungs. Similarly, introducing an allergen into the lungs of a person who has asthma but no hay fever unleashes inflammatory substances in the lungs and upper airways, including the nose and sinuses that are completely untouched by the allergen.

This close communication between the upper and lower airways is what scientists mean when they refer to asthma and allergies as being "one airway, one disease."

I think the concept helps explain some seemingly unrelated facts and figures: People with allergies are more prone to having problems with sinusitis, nasal polyps, ear infections and inflamed eyes. They tend to get bronchitis and pneumonia more easily. Those with eczema are susceptible to developing secondary bacterial infections of the skin.

In rare instances allergies can result in a life-threatening allergic reaction, called anaphylaxis. It usually occurs within minutes to an hour after exposure to an allergy-causing trigger. The reaction can cause constriction of the airways or a severely swollen tongue or throat. This can result in wheezing, great difficulty breathing, or even suffocation. The blood pressure may also suddenly drop and cause the person to pass out or go into shock. A medical emergency, anaphylaxis can lead to unconsciousness or death if treatment is not received right away.

Chapter 2
Diagnostic Steps

෬෩

Allergies are among the top ten reasons for health care visits. As we saw in the last chapter, they cause uncomfortable symptoms and may lead to a number of serious conditions. For these reasons, people with allergic disorders deserve to be carefully evaluated by a health professional, starting with a thorough medical history and physical examination.

Risk Factors

During your evaluation, your consulting physician may ask questions about your risk factors for allergies. The following factors are associated with an increased risk for developing an allergic disorder:

- Family history of eczema, hay fever, asthma or other allergies
- Personal history of eczema, hay fever, asthma or other allergies
- Male gender
- Firstborn status
- Birth during pollen season, usually in the spring or fall
- Birth by cesarean section
- Repeated use of antibiotics early in life

- Tobacco smoke exposure in the first year of life
- Exposure to toxic chemicals or pollutants
- Exposure to indoor allergens such as dust mites or pet dander

Diagnostic Tests

Depending on the results of your history and physical as well as your risk factors for allergies, further testing may be obtained to more fully assess possible allergic conditions. Options include skin and blood testing, which are employed for a variety of different allergic disorders, as well as breathing tests for asthma. The elimination diet and medically supervised food challenge are additional ways to acquire more data for evaluating possible food allergies.

Skin Testing

The test uses liquid preparations of allergy-causing agents like plant pollen, mold, house dust mite, pet dander, milk and wheat to test for allergies. In the test, drops of the different extracts are placed on your arm or back, and your skin underneath is pricked with a needle. Skin wheals or welts measuring more than three millimeters across indicate an allergic response. The test is considered the most sensitive and least expensive screening method for identifying specific causes of allergies. It's usually performed in the office of an allergy specialist, who may be equipped to treat an allergic reaction should one occur.

Blood Testing

Several types of blood tests can be performed to detect the presence or absence of allergies. Blood tests have the advantage of being safer and more convenient to perform than skin tests in the setting of a general medical office. Many of the blood tests check for antibodies. These proteins, which are produced by your white blood cells, act to identify and neutralize foreign objects like bacteria and viruses. The most important blood tests involve checking your blood for the amount of the allergic antibody, known as immunoglobulin E (IgE). When your body makes IgE to counteract allergy-causing substances, the antibody can be detected in your blood.

Total immunoglobulin E

A high level of total immunoglobulin E (total IgE) in your blood suggests the likelihood of allergies. If you have an allergic disorder like eczema or asthma, you may have an elevated total IgE. The test gives no conclusive proof of any condition, however, and does not reveal the cause of your allergies.

Allergen-specific immunoglobulin E

The presence and amount of antibodies to specific substances such as pollens or molds can be used to help diagnose allergies. These blood tests, called allergen-specific immunoglobulin E (IgE), are generally less accurate than skin tests. The accuracy averages only about 75 percent that of skin prick testing when looking at airborne allergies. Research suggests, however, that the two tests are roughly equivalent for the detection of certain food allergies.

Allergen-specific immunoglobulin G

Popular blood tests that measure immunoglobulin G (IgG) antibodies have not been validated scientifically. They are mostly performed for the evaluation of food allergies. According to research, the test results actually represent the body's normal immune responses to food, not true food allergies. For this reason, most allergy experts do not recommend relying on the tests for diagnostic purposes. But there is one exception. Studies indicate the tests are accurate for measuring a person's response to allergy shots that are given for insect venom allergies.

Asthma Tests

Breathing tests can be used to determine how much air moves in and out as you breathe. Spirometry measures how much air you can exhale in a short period of time. This can be done before and after taking an inhaled asthma medication, so the effect of the drug on your breathing can be measured. Improved airflow after inhaling the medication, which indicates the airway narrowing has reversed, is diagnostic of asthma.

Elimination Diet

An elimination diet can help you determine if certain foods are causing your symptoms or making them worse. It involves temporarily avoiding suspect foods and observing the results. Besides identifying possible food sensitivities and allergies, the diet can help you treat food-related symptoms. It should be done under the supervision of your health care provider.

Following is a brief overview of how an elimination diet is typically done. The diet often has four main phases.

Phase 1: Food diary

Start a diet journal and keep it for one week. Record every food and beverage you consume that week as well as the approximate amount, the date and the time. For any symptoms that you observe, write a description of how you felt and the symptom duration and time of onset.

Make a list of suspect foods to eliminate during the next phase of your diet. Some of the most common problem foods include dairy products such as cow's milk and butter, red meats, processed meats, eggs, wheat, corn, peanuts, pistachios, strawberries and citrus. Other likely culprits include processed foods, refined sugars, prepared condiments, margarine, shortening, alcohol, caffeinated beverages and sodas. Food additives such as sulfites and nitrites as well as artificial colors, flavors and preservatives are additional ingredients that sometimes bother people. Also be sure to notice foods you crave or eat a lot. Often these are the very foods that are creating sensitivities for you—albeit it in a counterintuitive manner.

Before moving on, I'd like to stress an important step that's often forgotten (at least, by my patients): Be sure to continue recording your observations in your food journal throughout all of the remaining phases of your elimination diet.

HEALTH TIP FROM DR. SMOOTS

Foods to Eat in an Elimination Diet

Question: What can I eat during an elimination diet?
Answer: After reading the list of common problem foods, you may wonder what's left for you to eat. Appendix A provides detailed examples of foods that are commonly allowed—as well as those to be avoided—during an elimination diet. I'll briefly summarize here. Typically, unless you notice a particular allergy or sensitivity, an elimination diet allows you to eat the following foods:

- Animal protein: Chicken, turkey, lamb, cold water fish
- Milk: Rice milk
- Legumes: Peas, lentils and all beans except soybeans and soy products

- Vegetables: All are allowed except corn and creamed vegetables
- Fruits: All are allowed except citrus and strawberries
- Grains and starches: Rice, millet, quinoa, amaranth, buckwheat, teff and potatoes. This includes breads and cereals made from these foods, and that are free of the ingredients you are trying to eliminate.
- Soups: Vegetable-based without thickening agents and not canned or creamed
- Beverages: Unsweetened fruit and vegetable juices, caffeine-free herbal teas, filtered or pure water
- Fats: Cold-pressed or expeller-pressed oils made from olive, canola or flax
- Nuts and seeds: Coconut, pine nuts, flax seeds
- Sweeteners: Brown rice syrup or fruit sweeteners

For more information: Please see Appendix A for more detailed food lists and explanations.

Phase 2: Food elimination

Eliminate your chosen foods for two weeks. Completely avoid eating the foods, either whole or as ingredients in other foods. To eliminate wheat from your diet, for example, you need to avoid all gluten-containing foods such as barley, rye, kamut, spelt and triticale. Also stay away from foods like oats that are often contaminated with wheat. In addition, eliminate food ingredients derived from wheat like gluten, malt, semolina and vegetable starch. Carefully read food labels and be cautious when dining out.

You may notice that your symptoms get worse for a day or two when you first begin the elimination diet. Consult your physician if your symptoms worsen more than briefly or become severe. Also check with your physician before proceeding onward if your symptoms did not improve during the elimination phase of your diet. You might need to go through phase two again, trying a couple of different elimination diets, before you are able to identify the problem foods.

Phase 3: Food challenge

If you noticed improvement during the elimination phase of your diet, you are ready to move on to the food challenge. During this phase you will again eat the eliminated foods one at a time. Begin by reintroducing a new food every three days. Eat the new food for one day, with small portions in the morning and larger portions in the afternoon and evening. Remove the new food after eating it for one day. Then wait two days to see if you notice any symptoms. If you develop a sudden or severe allergic reaction, seek medical care immediately.

The food probably is not a problem food if it doesn't cause symptoms during the challenge. You can add it back into your diet after you have finished testing all of the suspect foods on your list.

Phase 4: Long-term diet

The final step is to create a personalized diet based on the results of your elimination diet as well as input from your physician. To ensure you're getting adequate nutrition from your new diet, you should enlist the advice of your physician or ask for a referral to a dietician. A successful diet should help to keep your symptoms from coming back. If it doesn't, it's time to obtain additional professional advice about recurring or persisting problems.

Medically Supervised Food Challenge

The most accurate test for food allergies is the medically supervised food challenge. It is done to diagnose a food allergy or determine if your food allergy has resolved. During the test, you consume dried forms of the suspect foods in carefully controlled amounts. The test starts with a tiny amount of the food in question and then, if you have no reaction after a period of time, you may be given a slightly larger amount of the food. It is performed under the supervision of a health care professional who is trained to record and treat any reactions that you might have. A medically supervised food challenge may not be recommended if you're at risk for severe reactions.

Part II
Conventional Care of Allergic Conditions

ೞೞ

Chapter 3
Self Care

CR&O

You can do much to maintain your health and lessen the impact of your allergies with simple self care measures. Here are some practical steps you can take to get started on the road toward better health and more vibrant vitality. In the process you may likely notice that you are having fewer problems with your allergies.

Lifestyle Habits

Lifestyle habits that you hold day in and day out can dramatically affect your longevity and your health. When it comes to allergies, important areas to address include managing stress, getting sufficient sleep, exercising regularly, and achieving a healthy weight. The improvements you choose to make will have more lasting success if you take them one step at a time. Keep track of your progress and regularly reward yourself with a fun activity of your choosing such as movie night, enjoying a novel, or planning an outing with friends.

Rest & Relaxation

Too much stress has a damaging effect on your immune system. Research shows that impaired immunity can adversely impact nearly every part of your body from your head to your toes. It's no wonder, then, that asthma, eczema, hives and other allergic conditions often worsen when people experience more stress. Strong emotions and stressful events are well-known triggers of asthma attacks. To reduce stress:

- Get enough sleep. For most people this means seven to nine hours of restful slumber every night.
- Do something you enjoy every day, if possible, or at least a couple of times a week. Hobbies such as music, reading, journaling, puzzles, sketching or woodworking can bring needed stress relief.
- Talk to family members, significant others, or close friends who are supportive. Make a habit of participating in social activities with a group outside your immediate family at least once a month.
- Don't bring home your job-related problems or work. Manage your time at work efficiently and then shift gears to enjoy a change in scenery while you're at home. Also be sure to schedule regular vacations instead of rolling over your paid holiday leave.
- Talk to a health care professional if you're often using alcohol or other drugs for relaxation. Any addictive substance can be harmful to your health.
- Find a place in your home where you can relax and be by yourself. This is a good place to practice a relaxation technique from Chapter 12.
- Exercise for at least 30 minutes most days of the week to release stress. The next part of this chapter provides tips on how to get started.

Physical Activity

Regular exercise has a natural anti-inflammatory effect on your body that quiets allergies. It also helps to normalize the function of your immune system and quickly release stress.

Elizabeth Smoots MD

Gradually work up to at least 30 minutes of moderate exercise on five or more days each week. First get your physician's approval if you are unaccustomed to exercise, or plan to significantly increase your level of activity. Appendix B provides tips to help you stay motivated.

If you have asthma, regular exercise can strengthen your heart and your lungs. Greater cardiovascular health may also help alleviate troublesome asthma symptoms. Common-sense tips for exercising with asthma include:

- Warm up for 15 minutes and then gradually increase the intensity of your exercise.
- Avoid exercising in places that contain elevated levels of allergy-causing substances or polluted air.
- Avoid breathing cold air. When it's frigid outside, you can warm inhaled air by breathing through your nose and covering your nose and mouth with a scarf or face mask.
- Get a personalized exercise prescription from your provider that includes the frequency, intensity, duration and type of physical activity that you should be doing.
- Talk to your provider if your physical activities trigger asthma attacks. Making medication adjustments and changes in your exercise routine may help.

HEALTH TIP FROM DR. SMOOTS

Measures for Exercise-Induced Asthma

Some issues to consider and discuss with your physician, if you have exercise-induced asthma, include:

- In general, the physical activities most likely to exacerbate asthma are skiing, soccer, and long-distance running outdoors. Among the options less likely to be problematic are indoor swimming, tennis, baseball and basketball.

- Prescription medications such as albuterol and cromolyn sodium can help prevent exercise-induced asthma, when taken before physical activity. Chapter 6 has more information about these prescription medications.

- Scientific research shows that supplementing with fish oil daily can help alleviate exercise-induced breathing problems in asthma. Chapter 11 provides more information about taking fish oil.

- One small study of patients with exercise-induced asthma found that a large amount of vitamin C, a dose of 1,500 milligrams, taken before exercise, helped prevent airway narrowing and associated breathing problems during physical activity. See Chapter 11 for more information about vitamin C.

Healthy Weight

You probably know that excess weight is hazardous to your health. Fat cells produce hormones and chemicals that can have inflammatory effects on your body. Ongoing inflammation may worsen allergy and asthma symptoms and place you at higher risk for other health problems.

The good news is that you can significantly improve your health by losing only five to ten percent of your body weight. Talk to a health care professional about your barriers to weight loss. Some tips to help you get started toward a healthier weight and a fitter self include:

- Be your own expert. Create a dietary approach that works for you long-term. Lasting success often incorporates these simple principles: Consume a variety of foods. Avoid large meals that make you feel too full. Aim for a balance between eating for health and enjoyment.

- Listen to hunger signals. A growling stomach, loss of energy, headache, irritability and trouble concentrating are signs that your body may need to be nourished—if you pay attention to them. They will also let you know, based on when they go away, roughly when you have had enough to eat. When you learn to listen to the signals, hunger can help you decide when to eat and how much food is right for you.
- Find joy in exercise. Choose to do a physical activity you enjoy every day. Simple options include doing yard work, household chores, or parking and walking a little further. The previous section provides guidance about how to begin.
- Record your progress. Track your food intake, daily calories, and physical activities in a journal. The awareness you gain about your nutrition and activities can lead to wiser choices.

Home Remedies

Self care may involve using home remedies prepared from ingredients you have on hand or can buy inexpensively. Nasal saline irrigation and salt water gargles are good examples of popular home remedies for allergies.

Salt Water Gargles

Mix one-half teaspoon of salt in eight ounces of warm water and gargle several times a day. Spit out the water after gargling to avoid swallowing so much salt. The treatment may sooth bothersome throat irritation from persistent sinus drainage. It also helps break up the thick mucous threads of post-nasal congestion, the kind that sometimes keep dripping down the back of your throat.

Nasal Saline Irrigation

A nasal rinse can clear thick or excessive mucus from your nose. The procedure works well for unclogging stuffy nasal passages and helping sinuses to drain. It also flushes pollens or irritants from your nose before they trigger your allergies. In fact, several studies show the technique is more effective for hay fever, colds and sinus symptoms than over-the-counter medications.

To prepare for nasal saline irrigation, dissolve one teaspoon of non-iodized salt and one-half teaspoon of baking soda in 16 ounces of lukewarm water. For best results, use kosher, canning or pickling salt without additives. The water should be sterile or distilled. Tap water is acceptable only if it has been boiled for several minutes and then cooled, or if it's been passed through a filter with an absolute pore size of one micron or smaller. A note of warning: Do not use regular tap water for the nasal rinses. In rare instances, infections with the amoeba *Naegleria fowleri* have occurred in people who performed nasal irrigation with tap water. The amoebas can penetrate the nasal mucosa and invade the brain's membranes, where they may cause a fatal infection in susceptible people.

The next step is to perform the actual nasal saline irrigation. Fill a neti pot with some of the saline mixture. The pot has a long, tapered spout you can use to pour saline into your nasal cavities. While leaning over a bathroom sink, tilt your head to one side and place the pot's spout in your upper nostril. Slowly and gently pour the salt water into your upper

Elizabeth Smoots MD

nostril. The solution will run out your other nostril and the back of your throat. Spit out the drainage, gently blow your nose, and repeat on the other side. Continue the process until both sides of your nose are free of thick mucus. You can do the nasal rinses up to two or three times a day, if necessary. Rinse the neti pot after each use with distilled, sterile, or previously boiled and cooled water and let it air dry. Regularly sterilize your irrigation device at the end of the day to kill bacteria and mold.

Another alternative for irrigation is to purchase a commercially prepared sinus rinse kit. A number of companies make specially designed squeeze bottles that you can use in an upright position, with no tilting of your head required. The kits usually come with premixed saline solution, or salt packages for making it yourself. Several brands of nasal irrigators are also on the market. Carefully follow the manufacturer's directions.

Certain people should not do nasal irrigation. First check with your physician if you have a weak immune system, get frequent nosebleeds, find swallowing difficult, or have experienced nasal irritation or adverse effects from the procedure in the past. In addition, sinus irrigation is not recommended if you have blocked ears or are fighting an ear infection.

Health Care Savvy

Part of self care is to get the health care you need. In the case of hay fever, asthma, eczema or other allergies, scheduling regular health care visits can help you bring your condition under better control. Regular medical care also helps detect related non-allergic disorders earlier when they're easier to treat. Plus, being an active participant in your own care increases the quality of preventive and therapeutic recommendations you receive.

Non-Allergic Conditions

Certain health problems can aggravate allergies. It's not unusual for hay fever or asthma to flare, for example, if you are suffering from frequent viral infections or bouts of heartburn. The non-allergic disorders must be adequately addressed in these situations before you can gain lasting control of your allergy problems.

Viral infections

If you are someone who gets an allergy flare with every cold or flu, it's important to reduce your risk of contracting viral infections. The main prevention is to wash your hands frequently with soap and water. It takes at least 20 seconds to completely clean your hands. That's the amount of time it takes you to hum the "Happy Birthday" song from beginning to end twice.

Other ways to prevent colds and influenza can include: Limit your physical contact with others who are sick. Keep your hands away from your mouth, nose and eyes. And remember to get a flu shot every year.

Esophageal reflux

Heartburn is another condition that often aggravates allergies. The symptom consists of a burning sensation in your chest, usually behind your breast bone, that happens after meals. Heartburn usually occurs when the digestive acid in your stomach backs up into your throat. You may also notice a sour taste in your mouth from the backflow of your stomach contents.

Consult your physician if you experience heartburn frequently. Your physician can conduct an evaluation to determine whether or not you have the treatable condition gastroesophageal reflux. Left untreated, the disorder can potentially damage your airways and worsen asthma and allergy symptoms.

Health Care Participation

To receive the best possible medical care for your allergies and reduce disease risk, you need to take an active role in your health care team. Your team may consist of doctors, physician assistants, nurses, pharmacists and, most especially, you. With your participation, the whole team can function much better in meeting your health care needs.

As a member of your team, you will likely have certain responsibilities. For example, you may be expected to keep your team informed about your symptoms and all treatments and medicines that you're using. You may also be asked to help select from several treatment options based on your personal preferences and your understanding of the benefits and risks. Here are some additional tips for health care success:

Medication list

Tell your health care provider about all of your prescription and over-the-counter drugs as well as any herb or dietary supplements you are taking. Certain medications can contribute to the symptoms of asthma or allergies. Common culprits include beta blockers and non-steroidal anti-inflammatory drugs such as aspirin, ibuprofen and naproxen. Some people are allergic to particular medications such as penicillin or penicillin-based drugs. Over-the-counter cold and cough medications with multiple ingredients can be problematic for some people with allergies; talk to your physician or pharmacist for suggestions about which products are safest for you to use.

Asthma action plan

If you have asthma, talk to your physician about designing a personalized action plan. It's a written plan you develop with your doctor that can help you control your asthma. You can use the plan to track your medications and manage your symptoms. Typically, the plan describes how to handle worsening asthma symptoms or asthma attacks, and what to do in an emergency. You can also use it to treat ongoing lung inflammation, which may occur even if you are not having any symptoms, to minimize the long-term effects of asthma. The plan may include learning how to measure your peak expiratory flow with a peak flow meter. You can record your breathing measurements along with your symptoms and symptom triggers in a log. Schedule regular checkups with your physician to ensure your asthma action plan is working well for you. If it's not, you can get assistance from your health care team to help bring your symptoms under better control.

Emergency care

If you have severe allergies, you will need a plan for dealing with emergencies. Part of your plan should be to seek medical care immediately in case you experience a severe allergic reaction. Call 911 or the emergency phone number in your area. Other steps you can take, if you get bad reactions, are to wear a medical identification bracelet and carry epinephrine shots with you at all times. A medical alert necklace or bracelet lets others know about your allergy in case you have a reaction and cannot communicate. Giving yourself an epinephrine injection can help reduce your symptoms until you can obtain the emergency medical care you need. We will take a closer look at these lifesaving shots in Chapter 6.

Chapter 4
Avoidance of Triggers

ॐ

A trigger is anything that can set off your allergies. You may have a few or numerous allergy triggers. Airborne allergens like dust mites, pollen, cockroaches and animal dander are triggers for many people. So are foods such as peanuts, eggs, shellfish or food additives. In people with asthma, common triggers include viral respiratory infections, physical activity, and cold air. Latex or other substances you touch can cause allergic skin reactions. Other triggers include medications, insect stings, and menstrual cycles in some women.

It's well recognized that allergy triggers are different for different folks. To find yours, keep a record of your symptoms and the plants, animals, foods, chemicals or activities that seem to provoke them. Review your findings with your physician and ask what you can do. Once you've discovered the causes of your allergies, learning how to avoid the culprits is often the best treatment.

Following are avoidance strategies for some of the most common triggers that can bring about allergies.

Pollens

Pollens are the male fertilizing agents of flowering trees, grasses, weeds and other plants. The fine, powdery granules can easily become airborne. Pollen levels in the air are highest early in the morning and on hot, dry, windy days. To avoid pollen:

- Limit the time you spend outside between 5 a.m. and 10 a.m. This is when pollen is primarily emitted. Save outside activities for times of the day when pollen counts are lower, for example, in the late afternoon or after a heavy rain.

- Stay indoors on windy days when dust and pollen are blown around. Also limit your outside activities on hot, dry days, which tend to have very high pollen counts.

- Close windows and outside doors during pollen season. Your bedroom windows should be closed at night. Keep the windows of your car closed when you're out driving.

- Run the air conditioning in your house and car to reduce the amount of pollen that gains entry. Put allergy-grade filters in your air purifier or home ventilation system. Look into getting a high efficiency particulate air (HEPA) filter or electrostatic air filter, especially for your bedroom.

- Don't hang sheets and clothing out to dry as pollens and molds may collect on them. Instead, use a clothes dryer.

- Don't rake leaves, mow lawns, or be around freshly cut grass. Mowing and raking stirs up lots of pollens and molds. If you must do yard work or other outdoor activities, wear a dust mask.

Elizabeth Smoots MD

- Bathe or shower before bedtime to remove pollen and other allergens from your skin and hair.
- Go on vacation during the height of pollen season to a place with less pollen such as a desert or beach.

Dust Mites

Tiny microscopic relatives of the spider, house dust mites feed on the skin cells shed by pets and humans. Wastes produced by the mites are a major trigger of allergies and asthma. The mites thrive in the warm, humid environments commonly found in homes and are especially fond of carpets and soft furniture. To reduce the number of dust mites:

- Clean your home at least once a week. Vacuum and mop floors and vacuum carpets and soft furniture. Use a damp cloth to clean surfaces where dust can collect such as countertops, shelves and windows. Make sure to clean very thoroughly in your bedroom and other places where you spend a lot of time. Wear a mask while dusting or, better yet, have someone else do the cleaning for you.
- Consider getting a small particle or HEPA filter for your vacuum cleaner.
- Replace carpeting with hardwood or linoleum flooring if possible. Avoid or limit upholstered furniture, heavy draperies and soft toys that collect dust, especially in your bedroom.
- Wash all of your bedding in hot water once a week. Sheets, blankets, quilts and mattress pads must be cleaned in water heated to at least 130 degrees Fahrenheit in order to kill dust mites. Also wash your bed pillows every week, unless you put dust-proof covers on them.

- Use tightly woven, dust-proof covers on your mattress, box springs and pillows.
- Avoid wool or down blankets and feather pillows since they are difficult to clean, and some people are allergic to them. Likewise, use washable curtains and blinds.
- Keep the humidity in your home low by using a dehumidifier, especially if you live in a damp climate. Running an air conditioner is another way to lower indoor humidity and reduce your exposure to dust mites. You can also purchase special filters to help take circulating dust mites out of your home's air.

Molds

Molds are microscopic plants without stems, roots or leaves. Their spores float in the air like pollen. The growth of molds on fabrics, walls and other objects is called mildew. Indoor molds are found in attics, basements, bathrooms, shower curtains, refrigerators and garbage containers. Outdoor molds grow on decaying vegetation and rotting wood. To reduce your exposure to mold:

- Keep your home well ventilated and dry and maintain the humidity below 50 percent. Use a dehumidifier during humid weather. An air conditioner can help remove mold spores from the air. Change or clean heating and cooling system filters regularly.
- Limit the number of potted plants inside your house since molds like to grow on moist dirt.
- Regularly clean damp areas in your bathroom, kitchen and around the house to keep mold spores from forming. Use bleach to reduce mold growth on kitchen and bathroom surfaces.

Elizabeth Smoots MD

- Don't rake leaves or mow the lawn since these activities tend to stir up molds. Get rid of moldy leaves or damp firewood in your yard. If you're allergic to molds, have some else do these jobs for you. Wear a dust mask when you cannot avoid doing it yourself.

Cockroaches

These insects are pests that commonly invade our homes. Some of us develop allergies to cockroaches. Steps to rid your home of them include:

- Block cracks in the walls, ceilings and floors of your home where cockroaches can enter.
- Keep faucets and pipes in good repair so they do not leak.
- Promptly remove food waste from your house. Wash your dishes every day and take out the garbage. Do not leave food crumbs on your counters and floors. Clean them up promptly.
- Do not leave food or garbage in open containers. Store food, snacks and pet rations in sealed containers.
- Avoid chemical sprays to kill roaches since spraying can trigger asthma attacks. Carefully follow directions for poisons and traps and consider professional extermination.

Dander from Pets

Pets continually shed dead skin cells, or dander. The cells are light enough to be transported through the air, where they contribute to airborne allergies. To reduce pet dander in your home:

- Keep pets with fur or feathers out of your house, if you're allergic to dander. At the very least keep them out of your bedroom.
- Regularly bathe dogs and other pets when possible. Washing and brushing helps remove the dead skin cells. It also rinses away any pollen that stuck to their fur when they went outside. If you are not able to do it yourself, you can have your pet professionally bathed and groomed to reduce the dander in your home.
- Consider finding a new home for your pet. This is especially important if your symptoms are severe, or if an allergy to your pet is confirmed.
- Choose a pet without fur or feathers to eliminate the problem of dander. Some options include turtles, frogs, hermit crabs, fish, lizards and snakes.

Chemicals & Irritants

Some people are sensitive to strong odors, fumes and perfumes. Others find irritants like cigarette smoke or air pollution can set off their asthma or allergies. To reduce your exposure to toxins and chemicals:

- Make your home smoke-free. If you smoke cigarettes, talk to your physician about your options for quitting.
- Avoid cigarette smoke of all kinds in places where other people are smoking. Firsthand smoke consists of the particles and vapors that the smoker inhales directly, while secondhand smoke is that which is visibly exhaled by smokers and inhaled by others. In contrast, thirdhand smoke is the tarry residue that gets deposited in layers on walls, furniture and clothing; it then gets stirred up and released back into

the air. More than 250 poisonous toxins are contained in the various types of tobacco smoke.

- Eliminate aerosol sprays, perfumes, room deodorizers, cleaning products and other chemicals that can trigger your allergy symptoms.
- Minimize indoor air pollution. Don't char foods or use wood-burning stoves. Properly ventilate the fumes from paints, stains, varnishes and adhesives.
- Monitor your local air pollution levels. They are reported daily by the U.S. Environmental Protection Agency as the Air Quality Index.
- Protect yourself from air pollution. Stay indoors when pollution levels are high. Keep the windows closed and, if you have air conditioning, set it on "re-circulate." If you must go outside, breathe through your nose, avoid strenuous physical activities, and limit the time you spend outdoors.

HEALTH TIP FROM DR. SMOOTS

Air Pollution Safety

Are you looking for information about air pollution in your area? Every day the U.S. Environmental Protection Agency reports on local air pollution levels and provides maps of current conditions and daily forecasts. The levels of air pollution are graded using the Air Quality Index as follows:

- Good (0 to 50): Air quality is satisfactory and poses little or no health risk.
- Moderate (51 to 100): Pollution in this range may pose a moderate health concern for people who are unusually sensitive.

- Unhealthy for Sensitive Groups (101 to 150): Members of sensitive groups may experience health effects. People with heart disease or lung diseases such as asthma or emphysema are very vulnerable. So are children and older adults. In addition, people of all ages who exercise or work vigorously outdoors are at increased risk.
- Unhealthy (151 to 200): Everyone may begin to experience health effects; additionally, members of sensitive groups may experience more serious health effects.
- Very Unhealthy (201 to 300): Everyone may experience more serious health effects.
- Hazardous (301 to 500): This level triggers emergency health warnings about hazardous air conditions. The entire population is even more likely to be affected by serious health effects.

Along with publication of the Air Quality Index, the government provides guidelines about how to reduce your health risk from exposure to air pollution. For online information from the U.S. Environmental Protection Agency, go to *www.airnow.gov*.

Foods

Even a tiny amount of a food can trigger food allergies. The only way to prevent a reaction, since there's still no cure, is to stay away from problem foods. The most common culprits include milk, eggs, fish, shellfish, tree nuts, peanuts, wheat and soybeans. Food labels must list whether they contain these common food allergens. To avoid potentially serious reactions to foods:

- Always read the label before opening a package if you have food allergies. The official name of the major food allergen may appear in parenthesis right after the common name of the allergy source. Examples include enriched flour (wheat), casein (milk), and lecithin (soy). Sometimes a statement such as "Contains wheat, milk and soy" may appear immediately following or adjacent to the list of ingredients.
- Read a product's ingredient statement with each and every purchase. The manufacturer may change the ingredients listed on the label at any time.
- Remember that certain foods are not required to provide information on their label about allergy-causing ingredients. These include fresh fruits and vegetables, eggs, meat and poultry products, alcoholic beverages, and highly refined oils.
- Take extra precautions to avoid allergenic foods at restaurants and social gatherings. Many people don't understand that a small amount of food can cause a serious reaction. So don't eat food made by others when safety is in doubt.
- Educate those who prepare meals for you about how to avoid your food triggers. If you have severe food allergies, taking precautions when purchasing and cooking foods is especially important. Your food preparers must thoroughly wash their hands and clean surfaces that may have contacted problem foods in order to avoid triggering food allergies.

Chapter 5
Over-the-Counter Medications

CR∞

Your local pharmacy probably stocks many different nonprescription drugs for allergies. Get advice from your physician or a pharmacist before you buy them. Read the label and product instructions carefully and educate yourself about possible side effects. Check back with your physician if you have any questions or if side effects occur. Here is a description of some of the most popular over-the-counter allergy medications.

Saline Sprays

Nonprescription nasal salt water sprays moisten the inside of your nose. This can help prevent any crusting or buildup of mucus from blocking your nose and sinus openings. Saline solutions act to liquefy and clear your nasal secretions and reduce inflammation of your nasal passages. They also help keep the cilia in your nose active and healthy; these small hair-like structures lining your nasal passages beat with a sweeping action to remove bacteria and debris.

Additionally, salt solutions can rinse pollens and other allergens out of your nose at the end of the day. Some people use them to wash away mucus prior to using medicated nose sprays; this helps the medicines make better contact with inflamed membranes.

Several over-the-counter brands provide saline sprays in various sizes of squeeze bottles. Nonprescription kits are also commercially available for nasal saline irrigation; see the home remedies section of Chapter 3 for detailed information about this technique.

Antihistamines

These drugs block the action of a chemical in your body called histamine. In order to understand how antihistamines work, you need to know a bit about human physiology. When allergy-causing agents called allergens enter your body, they set off a chain of events that can result in the symptoms of allergies. Those allergens make contact with white blood cells in your body tissues. This incites the white blood cells to get busy and start producing specialized antibodies called immunoglobulin E (IgE). The antibodies then travel to mast cells, which are immune cells that specialize in producing histamine. The antibodies trigger the release of stored histamine from your mast cells. In the final step, histamine binds to cells around your body to cause the symptoms typical of allergy such as sneezing, watery eyes or wheezing.

Scientists have learned exactly where antihistamines work in this series of events. The drugs block the effect of histamine on the type H1 receptors of your body's cells. Histamine continues to be released, even when antihistamines are present, but does not produce allergy symptoms since the receptors of your body cells are blocked.

Antihistamines primarily function to reduce sneezing and running of your nose. The medications also help control itching of your nose, throat, skin and eyes. They do not, however, have much impact on decreasing nasal congestion like decongestants do.

Traditional Oral Antihistamines

First generation antihistamines include diphenhydramine (Benadryl), chlorpheniramine, hydroxyzine and others. They are not used as much anymore since they have numerous side effects. *Caution*: Traditional antihistamines are notorious for causing drowsiness and sedation. They can adversely affect concentration, coordination and driving performance and have been implicated in fatal motor vehicle accidents. The drugs may cause stimulation in children. Traditional antihistamines can also lead to dry eyes, dry mouth, trouble with urination, impotence and glaucoma.

Non-sedating Oral Antihistamines

Second and third generation oral antihistamines are less likely to make you feel drowsy. Medication names for the so-called "non-sedating antihistamines" include loratadine (Claritin), cetirizine (Zyrtec) and fexofenadine (Allegra). These drugs are popular choices for mild or intermittent symptoms of hay fever and allergies. *Caution*: Sedation can still occur, especially at higher doses. Dry eyes or other side effects may be a problem for some people.

Traditional Antihistamine Eye Drops

Several brands of antihistamine eye drops are available over-the-counter. The drops are typically used to treat mild allergic eye symptoms such as itching, burning, redness, tearing and sensitivity to light. Meant for short-term use, they have a rapid onset of action and may start working within a few minutes. Some over-the-counter products combine an antihistamine, such as naphazoline, with a drug that constricts arteries in the outer membranes of your eyes such as pheniramine (Naphcon-A, Visine-A). *Caution*: The eye drops can cause rebound redness and swelling if you use them for more than two weeks.

Newer Antihistamine Eye Drops

Scientists have developed newer types of antihistamines that can be applied in your eyes for longer-periods of time. Ketotifen (Alaway, Zaditor) is available as a nonprescription eye drop. As explained in more detail below, this particular medication also has mast-cell stabilizing properties. *Caution*: The drops may cause eye irritation or a flu-like syndrome. Do not use them to treat eye problems caused by contact lenses.

Decongestants

Decongestant drugs relieve stuffiness by constricting small blood vessels in your nasal mucosa. Their action helps relieve nasal congestion but not other types of allergy symptoms.

Oral Medications

Popular oral decongestants include pseudoephedrine and phenylephrine. They constrict the arteries in your nasal mucosa to reduce watery secretions and tissue swelling inside your nose. This results in less stuffiness and congestion of your nose and sinuses. Since decongestants do not relieve other types of allergy symptoms, they are often paired with antihistamines in combination pills. *Caution*: Decongestants have a number of adverse effects, including anxiety, irritability, insomnia, headache, and increased blood pressure and pulse. People who have high blood pressure or take monoamine oxidase inhibitors (usually used for depression) should not take them. Get your physician's approval before taking decongestants if you have cardiovascular disease, hyperthyroidism, prostate problems, or glaucoma.

Nasal Sprays

Phenylephrine (Neo-Synephrine) and oxymetazoline (Afrin) are among the leading decongestant nose sprays. They work quickly to relieve nasal stuffiness. They are not effective, however, for other types of allergy symptoms. *Caution*: Limit your use of decongestant nose sprays to three days. If you use them for a longer time, the sprays can cause rebound congestion and worsening symptoms when you stop them.

Mast Cell Stabilizers

These medications prevent the release of histamine from your mast cells. The immune cells produce and release histamine and other inflammatory chemicals that cause allergy symptoms such as sneezing, itchy eyes and wheezing. Unlike antihistamines, which block histamine's effects to stop allergy symptoms, mast cell stabilizers prevent the release of histamine in the first place.

Nasal Sprays

Cromolyn sodium (NasalCrom) is a nonprescritpion nasal spray that helps relieve hay fever symptoms. It acts to stabilize your mast cells and stop the release of histamine. You must use the nose spray several times a day to stabilize your mast cells and avoid the allergenic effects of histamine release. Cromolyn is most effective when you start it before your symptoms begin. You can initiate therapy approximately 30 minutes before you're exposed to an allergy trigger, for example, or a couple of weeks before the start of pollen season. It does not work as well once your allergy symptoms have already gotten out of hand. The medication is generally slow to start working; symptom improvement usually takes about two to four weeks.

Eye Drops

Some of the newer eye drops have antihistamine and mast-cell stabilizing activity. Ketotifen (Alaway, Zaditor) has both of these properties and is available without a prescription. It may be useful for frequent or persistent allergic eye conditions. *Caution*: The drops may cause eye irritation or a flu-like syndrome. Do not use them to treat eye problems caused by contact lenses.

Elizabeth Smoots MD

Chapter 6
Prescription Medications

CR&O

A number of prescription drugs are available for allergic rhinitis, eczema, asthma and other kinds of allergic conditions. Remember that prescriptions are powerful drugs that have side effects. To get the benefits you need while minimizing the risks, work closely with your health care provider. Tips for using medications wisely include:

Bring your medicine to every health care visit. Carry your medicine bottles in a bag. If you can't bring your actual medicine, then make a detailed list. Write down all the medicines you're taking, including dietary supplements, over-the-counter drugs and prescriptions.

Keep your provider informed about your health. Let your provider know about current and past medical disorders and treatments. Also inform your provider if you are pregnant or breastfeeding, or have any drug allergies.

Ask your provider questions about your medications. Learn the name of any new medicine and why you need to take it. How often should you take it? What are the side effects? If problems occur, who do you call? For a list of important questions, see "Medication Questions to Ask" below.

Find out how much the medication costs. If cost is a concern, ask your provider about less expensive options such as generic drugs. Also ask about non-drug treatments for your condition, including avoiding triggers, getting adequate exercise and rest, using simple self care techniques, and learning about the alternative therapies discussed later in this book.

Get to know your pharmacist. Fill all your prescriptions at the same drugstore. Ask about side effects and interactions with your other medicines. Make sure you have the right medicine and understand the directions before you leave.

Organize all of your medications at home. Use a pillbox to organize your medicine. Mark start and stop dates on your calendar. Pick up refills before you run out. Finally, don't share old medications with other people; instead, throw them out.

It's important to get started on the right foot when learning to take your medicines properly. In the next step we will take a look at some of the most important drugs prescribed for allergies.

HEALTH TIP FROM DR. SMOOTS

10 Medication Questions to Ask

Better doctor-patient communication has been shown to help prevent medication errors. To help ensure the safe and appropriate use of prescription drugs, you need to get all the information necessary to use your medicine correctly. Ask these 10 questions whenever medicines are part of your treatment plan.

1. What is the medicine called? Is it brand name or generic?

2. Why do I need to take the medicine? When can I stop?
3. How often and when do I take the medicine?
4. How exactly should I take the medicine? Should I avoid any foods, drinks, drugs, dietary supplements or activities while using this medicine?
5. How long will it take the medicine to start working?
6. What are the potential side effects? What do I do if they occur?
7. Does the medicine interact with any of my other medicine? Are there any over-the-counter drugs or dietary supplements I should not use while taking it?
8. Under what circumstances do I refill the medication?
9. Does the medicine require special storage?
10. Can you give me printed information about the medicine?

Antihistamines

These popular drugs block the action of histamine, a chemical released in your body during allergic reactions. Antihistamines alleviate symptoms such as sneezing, mucus production, and itching of your nose, throat and eyes. They are not effective for treating nasal congestion.

Oral Medications

Traditional oral antihistamines may make you feel tired or drowsy. Do not combine them with other sedating drugs. Newer non-sedating antihistamines are less likely to cause drowsiness, but sedation can still occur, especially at high doses. Since oral antihistamines do not relieve nasal congestion, they are sometimes combined with decongestant medications.

Nasal Sprays

The antihistamine nose sprays azelastine and olopatadine can alleviate the nasal symptoms of hay fever. They are prescribed for runny nose, sneezing and itching of the nose and throat. These second-generation antihistamines were developed to cause less drowsiness, but sedation may still occur. *Caution*: Do not combine them with alcohol or other sedatives and use caution when driving or operating machinery. Other potential side effects include a bitter taste, nasal ulcers, and nose bleeds.

Eye Drops

Antihistamine eye drops can help alleviate eye itchiness and irritation caused by allergies or hay fever. The drug names for prescription eye preparations include azelastine, olopatadine, bepotastine and epinastine. *Caution*: These drops may cause eye irritation or a flu-like syndrome. Do not use them to treat eye problems caused by contact lenses.

Mast Cell Stabilizers

Drugs in this class prevent the release of histamine from mast cells. Your body's mast cells produce and release histamine and other inflammatory chemicals that cause allergy symptoms such as sneezing, itchy eyes and wheezing. Unlike antihistamines, which block the action of histamine to stop allergy symptoms, mast cell stabilizers prevent the release of histamine in the first place.

Eye Drops

Some of the newer antihistamines have added mast-cell stabilizing activity. Drugs available as prescription eye drops that have both of these properties include nedocromil, alcaftadine and lodoxamide. Azelastine, olopatadine, bepotastine and epinastine are also in the same drug class. *Caution*: The eye drops may cause eye irritation or stinging, or a flu-like syndrome. Do not use them to treat eye problems caused by contact lenses.

Inhalers

Cromolyn is available as a hand-held inhaler in several countries outside of the United States. In the U.S., however, cromolyn is only available as a nebulizer solution for the treatment of asthma.

Nebulizers

Larger and less portable than inhalers, nebulizers are designed to deliver aerosolized therapy to patients with asthma. The mast cell stabilizer cromolyn sodium (Gastrocrom) comes as a solution for use in nebulizers. Not effective for the immediate relief of asthma attacks, cromolyn is usually prescribed for the long-term control of asthma. It also helps prevent exercise-induced asthma when used before physical activity. Cromolyn must be used regularly for two to four weeks to reach its full effect.

Anticholinergic Agents

Drugs in this class can reduce mucus secretions in your nose and lungs as well as other areas of your respiratory tract. The medications also help open up and relax constrictions in your airways.

Nasal Sprays

A prescription nasal spray called ipratropium bromide (Atrovent) has anticholinergic activity. It can alleviate severe running of your nose by stopping excess fluid production in your nasal glands. The spray is not effective for treating congestion, sneezing or postnasal drip. *Caution*: Side effects include nasal dryness, nosebleeds and sore throat. In rare instances, the drug can cause blurred vision, dizziness and trouble urinating. The medication is not recommended for people with glaucoma or prostate problems.

Inhalers

Ipratropium bromide (Atrovent HFA) is available as a lung inhaler. It acts to quickly relax your airways and make it easier for you to breathe. Prescribed mainly for emphysema and chronic bronchitis, it is sometimes used along with other medications to treat asthma attacks, including moderate to severe flare ups of asthma.

Corticosteroids

Corticosteroids are man-made versions of the natural human hormone cortisol. The drugs work to reduce or prevent swelling and inflammation in your body. Corticosteroids are commonly prescribed to treat allergic conditions and autoimmune disorders. They can also provide a source of hormones if your body's own cortisol becomes deficient. Corticosteroids have potent side effects and should only be taken under a doctor's careful supervision. Common adverse effects of the oral medication include weight gain, high blood sugar, heart and eye problems, and increased infections. The medicine can also cause growth problems in children, osteoporosis and other bone problems, changes in mood and thinking, and trouble sleeping. Corticosteroids are prescribed in a variety of different forms to combat allergies.

Nasal Sprays

Nasal corticosteroids are generally the most effective drugs for the long-term treatment of allergic rhinitis, or hay fever.

They can relieve sneezing, runny nose, itching of your mouth and nose, and postnasal drip. They're particularly efficacious for nasal congestion. In addition, the nasal sprays are often beneficial for helping control eye allergy symptoms like itching or tearing. The medication may take a few days or weeks to reach its full effect. *Caution*: Side effects include nose irritation or bleeding. The best preventive measures are to learn to use the nose spray properly and report problems promptly to your physician.

Eye Drops

Corticosteroid eye drops are sometimes prescribed for allergic eye conditions. The drops are usually reserved for severe disorders since they can have potentially sight-threatening side effects. *Caution*: Cataracts, glaucoma and worsening of viral eye infections are among the adverse effects that may occur. Treatment should be limited to one or two weeks and should be carefully monitored by an ophthalmologist.

Creams

Corticosteroid ointments, creams and lotions are commonly used treatments for eczema. They provide anti-inflammatory activity that can help reduce irritation, redness, itching and swelling of your skin. *Caution*: Adverse effects include skin thinning and stretch marks. The prescription medications need to be carefully monitored by your physician to avoid side effects.

Inhalers

Corticosteroid inhalers are often recommended for the long-term control of asthma. They function to decrease swelling and mucus production within your airways. Their anti-inflammatory action helps calm down symptoms and prevent asthma attacks. Corticosteroid inhalers are the primary drugs prescribed on a continual basis for chronic asthma management. You may need to use your inhaler for several days or weeks before you begin to experience the medication's maximum benefit. *Caution*: Potential side effects include sore throat, hoarseness, and fungal infections of the mouth. Delayed growth in children, osteoporosis, cataracts and glaucoma may also occur, especially at high doses.

Pills and Shots
Oral medications or injections into muscles or veins are the forms of corticosteroids most likely to cause side effects. They are generally saved for people with severe allergies. You may be prescribed these potent corticosteroids if you do not respond to other drugs or cannot tolerate them. The medications should only be taken under the close supervision of your physician. *Caution*: Adverse effects include weight gain, high blood sugar, heart and eye problems, and an increased risk of infections. The drugs can also cause growth problems in children, osteoporosis and other bone problems, changes in mood and thinking, and trouble sleeping. Since the side effects most commonly occur with long-term use, the medications are usually prescribed only for short periods of time.

Epinephrine

The common name for epinephrine is adrenaline. This well-known hormone acts to get your body ready for fighting or fleeing danger. It functions to open up your airways and make breathing easier. Other actions of the hormone include stimulating your heart, raising low blood pressure, and reducing swelling of your throat and lips. A synthetic form of epinephrine is available as an injection for emergencies such as serious allergic reactions or anaphylactic shock. Emergency rooms, urgent care centers, and medical clinics often stock a supply of these injections. Consumer versions (EpiPen, Twinject) are available for people with allergic reactions who need to carry the shots with them at all times.

If you have a history of severe allergic reactions to insect stings, foods, or other allergy-causing substances, talk to your physician about getting a prescription for the prefilled syringes. Make sure you receive instructions on how to correctly inject yourself with the medication. Find out when you should use the injections, and under what circumstances you should repeat them. Be prepared by keeping the injections on hand in case you ever need them. The epinephrine treatments can be lifesaving in an emergency.

Beta Agonists

After the natural human hormone adrenaline was discovered, scientists modified the molecule to produce beta agonist drugs for asthma. These medications have since been further refined to act mainly on your lungs and less on your heart. The most selective beta agonist drugs dilate the airways of your lungs without increasing your blood pressure or pulse very much.

Inhalers

Inhaled beta agonists come in both short-acting and long-acting forms. The short-acting inhalers are a mainstay of acute asthma therapy. Also known as "rescue inhalers," they work quickly to dilate your bronchioles and ease wheezing and shortness of breath during an asthma attack. When used before physical activity, they may help prevent exercise-induced asthma. Popular drug names include albuterol and pirbuterol. Long-acting inhalers may play a role in the long-term control of moderate to severe asthma along with other medications. Salmeterol and formoterol are some of the most widely prescribed long-acting drugs. *Caution*: The most common side effects of beta agonist drugs are tremors and rapid heartbeat. Long-acting beta agonist inhalers may mask the deterioration of asthma; they should not be used to treat an acute asthma attack, and never should be used as a sole medication.

Pills and Shots
When an inhaler cannot be used, short-acting beta agonist drugs can be given orally or as an injection for the acute treatment of severe flares of asthma. The risk of adverse effects is higher with these formulations than with the asthma inhalers.

Leukotriene Modifiers

Leukotrienes are natural substances produced in your body as part of the allergic response. These chemicals can contribute to nasal congestion in hay fever as well as mucus production and airway narrowing in asthma. Scientists have developed oral medications that can reduce leukotriene levels in your body. These leukotriene modifiers include montelukast (Singular), zafirlukast (Accolate) and zileuton (Zyflo). They are primarily used to treat asthma. Only montelukast has been approved for the treatment of hay fever. *Caution*: Side effects include headaches, insomnia, anxiety, depression and suicidal behavior. Seek medical advice right away if you experience any adverse effects.

Antibody Neutralizers

Special antibodies called immunoglobulin E (IgE) play a central role in allergic disorders. The antibodies bind to your mast cells and release the chemical histamine that triggers sneezing and other allergic symptoms. Scientists have created a drug that binds to immunoglobin E in your body to neutralize its allergenic effect. The medication, omalizumab (Xolair), must be given by injection every two to four weeks. It is sometimes prescribed for people with moderate to severe allergic asthma not controlled by other medications. *Caution*: Severe allergic reactions or anaphylaxis to the medication have occurred. The injections must be given in a medical setting where trained personnel can monitor and treat any adverse reactions. Other side effects include headaches and redness or swelling of the injection site.

Chapter 7
Immunotherapy

CR&O

If medications don't control your symptoms, or cause too many side effects, you may be referred to an allergist to discuss allergy shots. Immunotherapy and desensitization therapy are other terms for the popular treatment. The process consists of gradually getting increasing amounts of allergy-causing substances to help you become less sensitive to them over time. This approach helps your body become accustomed to the allergens so you tolerate them better with fewer distressing symptoms.

While the mechanism of action is not fully understood, research shows that immunotherapy alters the way your body's immune system responds to potential allergens. Studies have documented changes in the production of inflammatory chemicals, allergic antibodies, and some types of immune cells.

Immunotherapy is usually given by injection in the U.S. But interest is growing in emerging treatments that involve taking the allergens orally or under the tongue.

Allergy Shots

The medical term for allergy shots is subcutaneous immunotherapy. It consists of injecting tiny amounts of allergens under your skin. As you build tolerance to them, the amounts of allergens in your injections are gradually increased over time. The injections are initially given one to three times per week during a build up phase that lasts for a couple of months. During the maintenance phase of subcutaneous immunotherapy, the injections are given every two to four weeks for a total treatment period of at least three to five years.

The injections are most effective for allergies to trees, grasses, weeds, dander from pets, dust mites, molds and cockroaches. Allergy shots are also used in the treatment of allergies to certain types of stinging insects such as bees, wasps, hornets and ants.

An extensive body of evidence indicates that subcutaneous immunotherapy is effective in the treatment of hay fever, eye allergies, and allergic asthma in both children and adults. People with both hay fever and asthma can gain particular benefit. In children, allergy shots may help prevent the progression of eye allergies or hay fever to allergic asthma. A study of 147 people showed those who received allergy shots as children cut their risk of developing asthma nearly in half.

You may want to consider consulting with a physician about allergy shots if you:

- Have failed to get symptom relief from drugs
- Have had unacceptable side effects
- Want to reduce or avoid the long-term use of medication
- Have both hay fever and asthma
- Want to prevent asthma in a child who has eye allergies or hay fever

Elizabeth Smoots MD

The injections are usually given in a medical office setting with health professionals on hand to observe and treat any adverse reactions that might occur. Mild side effects from the allergy shots can consist of redness or swelling at the injection site, while severe reactions include trouble breathing or anaphylactic shock.

Emerging Treatments

Allergy shots are the established form of immunotherapy in the U.S. However, oral immunotherapy and sublingual immunotherapy are emerging treatments that are gaining greater acceptance among conventional allergists in the U.S. and in other parts of the world.

Sublingual Immunotherapy

In this treatment tiny amounts of allergens are placed under your tongue instead of being given by injection. A dissolvable tablet or liquid extract is usually held in your mouth for a few minutes and then swallowed. Immune tissue in your throat and intestines responds to the allergens in the tablet in such a way that your tolerance to the allergens improves. Over a period of three to five years the method seems to decrease sensitivity to allergies in much the same way as do the injections.

Compared to allergy shots, however, the sublingual method avoids the need for injections and has a lower risk of severe side effects such as anaphylaxis. Adverse effects that may occur include gastrointestinal upset and itching or swelling of the mouth.

The effectiveness of sublingual immunotherapy has been demonstrated in children and adults in high quality studies in the U.S. and Europe. This therapy has been approved and widely employed in many areas of Europe. But the tablets and allergy extracts used in the treatment are not closely regulated in the U.S. and have not been approved by the U.S. Food and Drug Administration.

Oral Immunotherapy

This therapy is similar to sublingual immunotherapy but involves swallowing tiny amounts of allergens instead of putting them under your tongue. Enteric-coated tablets are used so the allergens can pass through your stomach undisturbed. The medicine usually dissolves in your small intestines, where it interacts with your lymph nodes and other immune tissues to create greater tolerance to allergies.

Elizabeth Smoots MD

Part III
Alternative Therapies for Allergic Conditions

৪৩৫৪

Chapter 8
Nutrition

✺

Despite little recognition of diet in conventional medical care, what you put in your mouth can have a noticeable impact on your allergies. That's good news since nutrition is largely under your control. You, or the people who prepare food for you, have an opportunity to make choices that influence your health every time you shop, prepare food and eat.

Here are some simple dietary modifications you can make to help improve the balance of allergy-inhibiting and allergy-promoting substances in your body.

Dietary Protein

Excess protein in your diet can irritate your immune system. While it's necessary to consume adequate amounts of protein for good health, consuming more than you need has a tendency to rev up your immune system. Eating one or two high-protein meals probably won't make a difference, but continuing to eat surplus protein on a regular basis can keep your system in a state of high alert.

To calm down your allergies, avoid routinely consuming large amounts of high-protein foods. These include sources of animal protein like meat, poultry and eggs as well as plant protein like beans, seeds and nuts. Studies indicate, however, that excess animal protein is much more inflammatory to the immune system compared to plant sources. So make a point of limiting animal protein in your diet for the greatest effect.

Dairy Products

Scientific studies have yet to find conclusive evidence that dairy intake worsens allergies. But I have long observed in my patients, my friends, and myself that dairy products trigger more mucus in the nasal passages, sinuses and airways.

The main cause of the increased mucus is the protein in cow's milk. Casein and other proteins in the milk appear to have irritating effects on the immune systems of certain sensitive individuals.

While not everyone is affected, those with a genetic predisposition seem to have a greater sensitivity to milk. This is not a true milk allergy and is not the same as milk intolerance, in which ingesting milk causes digestive ills. Some allergic people are just plain sensitive to the mucus-causing properties of milk.

What can you do about it? The best course of action I've found is to minimize or eliminate your use of milk and dairy products. Even cheese and yogurt can eventually lead to problems with "milk mucus." Read labels and avoid all foods listing milk as an ingredient.

It is often helpful to totally eliminate dairy products for six to eight weeks. Observe and record your symptoms in a journal during this time. Many allergy sufferers notice a dramatic improvement in their mucus production after eliminating milk for two months.

A dairy-free diet has its challenges since milk is such a common ingredient. Fortunately, there are many cow's milk substitutes on the market. I usually purchase soy milk and

Elizabeth Smoots MD

enjoy almond milk on occasion. Other people prefer milks made from grains such as rice or oats. In addition, substitutes for cheese and yogurt are readily available. Read labels carefully, however, and avoid products with added casein.

Calcium deficiency is a risk if you are eliminating dairy products. You will need to make an effort to get sufficient calcium from non-dairy foods such as greens, beans, seeds and canned fish. Milk and dairy substitutes are usually good sources of calcium, too. See Appendices C and D for a list of calcium-rich foods, and how to find out how much calcium you're getting.

Eventually, some people with milk sensitivity may get to the place where they can tolerate occasional consumption of small amounts of dairy products. This is something that people with true milk allergy cannot do.

Healthy & Unhealthy Fats

When it comes to allergies, not all fats are created equal. Research suggests that omega-3 fats may calm down inflammation and allergic disorders. Conversely, trans fats can trigger inflammatory and allergic conditions as can saturated fats and omega-6 fatty acids.

Anti-inflammatory Fats

The omega-3 fats found in seafood and some plants are essential for good health. Your diet is the only source since your body cannot make omega-3 fatty acids. Most people are deficient since they eat little or no fish or other omega-3 sources.

A deficiency is further compounded by consuming lots of omega-6 fats found in processed foods and vegetable oils. The ratio of omega-6 fats to omega-3 fats in the U.S. population averages eleven to one, even though the ratio recommended by nutrition experts is four to one or less.

An excellent way to restore a healthier balance of dietary fats is to eat more fish or take fish oil supplements. The omega-3 fats have anti-inflammatory effects that help reduce swelling and excess mucus in your nose and sinuses to bring allergy relief. Eating at least two servings of seafood every week is generally recommended. Fatty, cold-water fish like salmon, sardines, herring, mackerel, tuna and trout are especially rich in omega-3 fatty acids. Chapter 11 provides answers to your questions about taking fish oil.

What to do if you don't consume fish or fish oil? Vegetarians and people who dislike fish can obtain omega-3 fats from plant sources. Flax seeds contain them in abundant supply. I usually recommend one to two tablespoons of ground flax seeds per day. Since ground flax goes rancid rapidly, grind the seeds fresh daily in a coffee grinder or small blender. Other plant sources of omega-3 fats include walnuts, hemp seeds, canola oil, and soy products. Although soy oil is a good source of omega-3 fats, it is not recommended since it contains large amounts of omega-6 fats.

Keep in mind that your body uses omega-3s from plants much less efficiently than those found in fish. Only about four percent of the plant precursor alpha-linolenic acid can be converted into usable omega-3 fatty acids by the human body.

Overall, the healthiest oils for people with allergies are found in fish and flax seeds. The natural oils in nuts, seeds, avocados and extra-virgin olive oil also have anti-inflammatory effects.

Healthy Seafood Choices

You can get online information about making healthy seafood choices at the following websites:

- U.S. Food and Drug Administration, *www.fda.gov/food*
- U.S. Environmental Protection Agency, *www.epa.gov*
- Environmental Defense Fund, *www.edf.org/oceans*
- Blue Ocean Institute, *www.blueocean.org*
- Institute for Agriculture and Trade Policy, *www.iatp.org*
- Monterey Bay Aquarium, *www.montereybayaquarium.org*

Inflammatory Fats

On the flip side are certain fats that can potentially worsen inflammation and allergies. A major culprit, trans fat, is synthesized and added to many processed and convenience foods to improve their shelf life. It's important to keep your intake of trans fatty acids as close to zero as possible. To find out if trans fats are present in a food product, look for the words "partially hydrogenated oil" on the list of ingredients.

Be aware that U.S. laws have made it permissible to have misleading labeling when it comes to trans fats. Foods that claim to be "trans fat free" or to have "zero trans fats" may still contain as much as 0.5 grams of trans fats per serving. These undeclared grams can add up if you have more than one serving or eat multiple processed foods that contain trans fat.

Omega-6 fatty acids are another group of fats that can contribute to a downward allergy spiral. As discussed above, the omega-6 fats in processed foods and vegetable oils can worsen an already existing omega-3 fat deficiency. Excessive amounts of omega-6 fatty acids stimulate an inflammatory response in the body that can aggravate allergies. Restrict your consumption of polyunsaturated vegetable oils such as sunflower, safflower, corn, cottonseed and soybean since these oils contain omega-6 fats in large amounts.

Last are the saturated fats. They are found in fatty meats, chicken with the skin, dairy products, coconut oil, and palm oil. Research indicates that consumption of large amounts of saturated fats may initiate or aggravate inflammation in your body. The U.S. government advises keeping the consumption of saturated fats to less than 10 percent of daily calories. The American Heart Association has a more stringent limit, recommending that fewer than seven percent of your daily calories come from saturated fat. No danger exists in restricting saturated fats in your diet since your body can make all it needs from other foods.

In summary, the evidence suggests that trans fats in particular, and omega-6 fats and saturated fats to a lesser degree, can promote inflammation in your body. It is wise to limit your use of pro-inflammatory fats to avoid having them worsen your allergies.

Anti-inflammatory Diet

Next in the lineup of nutritional changes that calm allergic disease is the anti-inflammatory diet. The process of inflammation helps your body perform vital functions like fighting infections and repairing wounds. But when the protective process doesn't turn off, it can lead to harmful effects in the form of chronic diseases like allergies and asthma. Different foods contain substances that can directly promote or inhibit your body's production of chemicals that lead to persistent inflammation.

For this reason, people with allergic disorders often receive a great deal of benefit from an anti-inflammatory diet. The diet can help you start eating more foods that reduce inflammation, while consuming fewer foods that increase inflammation. This eating pattern helps control the kind of chronic, low-level inflammation that contributes to allergies.

The anti-inflammatory diet emphasizes antioxidant-rich fruits and vegetables, legumes and seafood while limiting refined flours, sugar, unhealthy fats, and animal protein in excessive amounts. The following version of the anti-inflammatory diet has been popularized by Andrew Weil, MD, founder and director of the Arizona Center for Integrative Medicine at the University of Arizona, where I completed my fellowship in integrative medicine. I regularly use this diet in my practice and at home.

Fruits
Eat three to four servings of fruit every day in a wide range of colors. One serving consists of a medium piece of fruit, half a cup of chopped fresh or frozen fruit, or a quarter cup of dried fruit. Choose organic whenever possible. Appendices E and F provide lists of the fruits and vegetables most likely—and least likely—to be contaminated with pesticides, respectively.

Vegetables
A minimum of four to five servings of vegetables a day is recommended. One serving equals a half cup of cut-up raw or cooked vegetables or a cup of raw leafy greens. Organic vegetables in a rainbow of colors are preferred. See Appendices E and F for the "Dirty Dozen" and "Clean Fifteen" when it comes to vegetables and fruit.

Grains, Pasta & Beans

The anti-inflammatory diet recommends one to two daily servings of beans, three to five daily servings of whole or cracked grains, and two to three weekly servings of pasta. For each, a serving is a half cup cooked. The pasta is lightly cooked so it still has some tooth, also called "al dente."

The term "whole grains" in this diet refers to grains that are intact or in a few large pieces, as opposed to products made from flour. These larger pieces digest more slowly than do bread, bagels, tortillas and other products made from whole wheat flour or refined white flour. Slower digestion reduces the size and frequency of blood sugar spikes that can promote inflammation.

Fats

Healthy fats such as olive oil, canola oil, nuts, avocados and seeds are recommended, about five to seven servings a day. A serving of oil is one teaspoon. Walnuts, flaxseeds, and oily fish are especially good sources of omega-3 fats, known to have anti-inflammatory effects. Reduce your intake of pro-inflammatory fats as described in the preceding section on fats.

Proteins

Try to get less protein from animal sources and more from vegetable sources such as beans and soy products. Good protein sources include soy foods, one to two servings a day, and seafood, two to six servings a week. Other types of animal protein such as lean meats, skinless poultry, dairy products, and eggs are limited to one to two servings a week. A serving is equal to a half cup of tofu or edamame, one cup of soymilk, one ounce of cheese, eight ounces of dairy, one egg, or three ounces of cooked fish or meat.

Elizabeth Smoots MD

Cooked Asian Mushrooms

Known to enhance immune function, cooked Asian mushrooms are allowed in unlimited amounts. Some common examples are shiitake, maitake, enoki, and oyster mushrooms. Limit your consumption of common commercial mushrooms, including button, crimini and portobello, since they contain natural carcinogens that are only partly deactivated even when they're quite well cooked.

Healthy Herbs & Spices

Turmeric, ginger, garlic, rosemary and other spices are encouraged in unlimited amounts for seasoning your food. Most of the herbs and spices commonly employed in cooking have powerful antioxidant and anti-inflammatory properties.

Tea

Drink white, green or oolong varieties of tea, two to four cups per day. These varieties of tea are especially rich in a group of antioxidant compounds called catechins that reduce inflammation.

Red Wine

Red wine is considered optional. Drink no more than one to two glasses a day. It is not recommended if you do not already drink alcohol since overuse of the beverage has potential adverse effects.

Healthy Sweets

Healthful dessert choices can be enjoyed sparingly. Options include unsweetened dried fruit, dark chocolate containing at least 70 percent cocoa, and fruit sorbet. Sugary foods in larger amounts can cause blood sugar spikes in your body that tend to worsen inflammation.

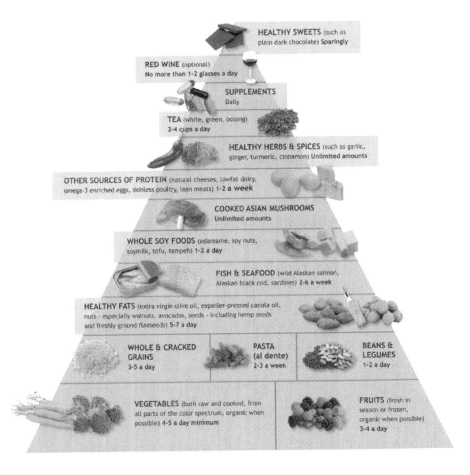

The Anti-Inflammatory Diet Pyramid
Courtesy of drweil.com, Weil Lifestyle, LLC

Elizabeth Smoots MD

Low-Glycemic Diet

Both sugar and refined flour have a high glycemic index, a term coined by researchers at the University of Sydney in Australia to describe foods that create rapid ups and downs in blood sugar after eating. The speed at which a carbohydrate raises blood sugar relates to its chemical structure, the food's surface area available for digestion, and the presence of fiber or fat.

In the rating system, each food is compared with the effects of pure glucose (rated 100). Foods with a high glycemic index (more than 70) are digested quickly, providing you with fast burst of energy followed by an energy drop. On the other hand, low-glycemic foods, those with a glycemic index less than 55, release energy slowly over a longer period of time. The rate of glucose absorption is the main determinant of how healthful or harmful a carbohydrate is for your health.

A rapid rise and fall in your blood sugar is inflammatory and can aggravate allergies when it occurs repetitively in your body. To control inflammation you should avoid or limit foods that create large blood sugar spikes.

HEALTH TIP FROM DR. SMOOTS

Low-Glycemic Diet Resources

A book written by Jennie Brand-Miller, PhD, and Kaye Foster-Powell, *The New Glucose Revolution*, provides detailed information about eating a low-glycemic diet. Also available is a concise version, *The New Glucose Revolution Pocket Guide to the Top 100 Glycemic Foods*. In addition, you can view the

University of Sydney's Glycemic Index Database at *www.glycemicindex.com*.

Food Allergies & Sensitivities

Food allergies or sensitivities can contribute to hay fever, asthma, eczema and other allergic conditions, as discussed in Chapter 1. Going on an elimination diet for a few weeks is a good way to tease out whether or not you are experiencing allergies or sensitivities to food. The diet can also help you discover if food additives such as sulfites and nitrites as well as artificial colors, flavors and preservatives are aggravating your symptoms. A food challenge often follows the elimination diet. Keeping a diary of the foods you eat and your symptoms when you do, or do not, eat them can provide useful information about possible sensitivities. See Chapter 2 for information about how to do an elimination diet and food challenge. I have provided guidance about how to avoid or minimize contact with food allergy triggers in Chapter 4.

Chapter 9
Aromatherapy & Essential Oils

CREBO

You can probably recognize the distinctive smell of peppermint or rosemary. But did you know the volatile oils of these and many other plants have therapeutic effects? Fragrant essential oils derived from plants have a very rich history in Egypt, Greece, the Middle East, India, Asia and countless other areas of the world. They have gained popularity in modern times as awareness of their medicinal value has grown.

You can use them several ways to support your health and thwart disease. Aromatherapy is a technique that involves aerosolizing essential oils with a diffuser, steam inhalation or bath to make them available for inhalation. Dilute amounts of essential oils can be applied to your skin for treating some conditions. A few essential oils are even taken by mouth with proper supervision and care. The various treatment methods are thought to supply your body with plant substances in therapeutic amounts.

The highest quality essential oils on the market today are extracted from plants by steam distillation. A fairly new method using hypercritical carbon dioxide may also yield superior oils. Lower-quality products are also commonly available. For health purposes, avoid inferior oils that are extracted with chemical solvents or that use synthetic fragrances or artificial ingredients.

Safety precautions are necessary since essential oils are usually produced in highly concentrated forms. Avoid getting the oils or their strong vapors in your eyes. Always dilute essential oils in a carrier such as almond, canola, olive or sesame oil before applying them to your skin. Only take essential oils by mouth with appropriate medical supervision since many are toxic when consumed. Vary the essential oils you use regularly. And keep essential oils out of the reach of young children.

You can do a patch test to determine if you are sensitive to a particular essential oil. To do this, dilute 10 drops of essential oil in one ounce of a carrier such as canola, soy or safflower oil. Rub a bit of the oil into a small patch of skin at the crook of your arm or the front of your chest. Then check the area in 12 hours for any signs of skin irritation, redness or itching.

Despite its reputation as a natural treatment, aromatherapy can still have adverse effects. Reports have been issued of essential oils causing allergic reactions, increased sensitivity to sunlight, seizures, kidney failure and other toxic effects. The risks are much higher when the oils are consumed as opposed to inhaled or applied topically.

As a precaution, people at risk for harm should only take essential oils under the supervision of a physician. Especially vulnerable are pregnant or nursing women, children, and people with kidney or liver disease or other chronic illnesses.

Inhalation of Essential Oils

People the world over most often inhale essential oils to support wellness or treat disease. This method of delivery is called aromatherapy. It involves aerosolizing the essential oils using a diffuser, humidifier, inhaler, steam inhalation or bath, and then inhaling the vapors.

A variety of diffusers and humidifiers are available on the market. Or you can make your own steam inhalation or bath very simply. To prepare a bath, put three to ten drops of the desired essential oil in a tub full of warm water. Relax and enjoy the scent as you bathe.

For a steam inhalation that you can create in your own home, start out by bringing a pot of water to a boil. Carefully pour the boiling water into a large heavy bowl. Add three to ten drops of the essential oil. Sit down in front of the bowl and lean forward, holding your face at least a foot away from the hot water. Drape a towel over your head to contain the steam in a makeshift tent as you breathe deeply. Keep your eyes closed the entire time to avoid eye irritation. Continue to inhale the vapors through your nose for about 10 to 15 minutes. Don't use a steam inhalation during an asthma attack since the treatment may potentially worsen asthma symptoms.

Peppermint (*Mentha piperita*)

You can use essential oil of peppermint in a steam inhalation, bath or vaporizer. The therapy usually has a cooling effect on the body. Peppermint's properties may help relieve mucous congestion of your nasal passages, sinuses and lungs. Breathing the essential oil vapors often provides benefit for coughs and colds as well as congestion caused by allergies. *Caution*: When taken by mouth, peppermint can worsen symptoms of heartburn or esophageal reflux. Do not apply peppermint oil on the faces of children under five years since it may impair breathing.

Eucalyptus (*Eucalyptus globulus*)

Research indicates that eucalyptus essential oil exerts beneficial effects on respiratory infections such as colds, coughs, sinusitis and bronchitis. It is also used as a remedy for asthma. Besides having a cooling effect on your body, the essential oil can help diminish inflammation and dilate airways in your lungs. It acts as an expectorant to help thin and remove mucus from your respiratory tract. Eucalyptus essential oil can relieve cough and improve breathing. Additionally, it has antibacterial and antiviral activity.

Thyme (*Thymus vulgaris*)

The substance thymol in this aromatic essential oil provides a natural treatment for upper respiratory tract infections. The herb can help calm coughs, relieve congestion, reduce inflammation, and support your body in fighting the underlying viral infection. In addition, thyme has the ability to thin and expel phlegm in children and adults with copious mucus production related to colds, bronchitis, sinusitis, allergies or asthma.

Marjoram (*Origanum marjorana*)

The essential oil of the household herb marjoram may have a warming effect on your body. Marjoram reduces inflammation and breaks up congestion. Vapors from the essential oil can also help ease your breathing. The herb has significant antimicrobial activity that can help fight viral infections such as colds, influenza and laryngitis.

Rosemary (*Rosmarinus officinalis*)

Rosemary has been employed as an antiseptic and food preservative since ancient times. Research shows the herb has antibacterial activity. Its decongestant properties often prove valuable for respiratory conditions. You can use essential oil of rosemary to help clear your nose and sinuses, decrease lung congestion, and improve your breathing.

Myrtle (*Myrtus communis*)

The essential oil of myrtle is known for its calming and respiratory effects. Its activity can help alleviate congestion of your nasal passages, sinuses and lungs. The essential oil is often used in a steam inhalation to calm down coughing and encourage better breathing. Myrtle also works to reduce inflammation and ward off bacteria, making it valuable in the treatment of lung and respiratory infections.

Topical Use of Essential Oils

Essential oils can be diluted in oil and applied to your skin for certain health conditions. Since they are so concentrated, in most cases they should not be used on your skin in undiluted form. A few drops of an appropriate essential oil are usually added to a larger quantity of carrier oil. When dilute formulations of essential oils are rubbed on your chest and back, they are absorbed into your skin and chest while the aromatic vapors are inhaled into your lungs.

Vapor Rub

Products such as Vicks VapoRub contain the essential oils of peppermint, eucalyptus and camphor in a gel base. Rubbing the gel on your chest, throat and back may help relieve symptoms of an upper respiratory infection such as cough or congestion of your nose or chest. Sometimes the products are used to open up stuffy nasal passages and congested sinuses associated with allergies, though any improvements are usually temporary. *Typical dosage*: Follow product directions carefully. *Caution:* Avoid contact with your eyes, nostrils, mouth or areas of damaged skin. Application of the gel on your chest, throat, back or other areas can cause local skin irritation. It may also cause watery eyes and a burning sensation of your nose and lips.

Calendula (*Calendula officinalis*)

The name of the ornamental pot marigold comes from its ability to bloom nearly around the calendar, from early spring to first frost. Its flowers have been used medicinally since ancient times to treat inflamed skin and seal over wounds. Research shows the flowers have anti-inflammatory properties that relieve minor skin conditions and significantly speed up wound healing. Widely available in the U.S. and around the world, calendula creams and ointments are often used to treat allergic skin conditions such as eczema. The skin care products are prepared in a variety of different ways. Traditionally made from alcohol extracts or herb-infused oils, they are also available as essential oils incorporated into a cream base. *Typical dosage*: Apply the cream or ointment to affected areas of skin three or four times a day. *Caution*: People with allergies to daisies may also be allergic to calendula. The herb may potentially interact with sedatives or blood pressure medications.

Chamomile (*Matricaria recutita*)

Chamomile flowers are a favorite of mine for treating stomach upset and nervous tension. They are also a good remedy for skin problems such as eczema. Chamomile creams are prepared from essential oils, alcohol extracts, or herb-infused oils that are incorporated into emollient creams or ointments. Scientists have found these topical chamomile formulations are as effective as low-potency hydrocortisone creams. The herb has a minimal risk of side effects, making it ideal for daily skin care. *Typical dosage*: Follow product directions for commercially prepared chamomile creams. *Caution*: In rare circumstances, allergic reactions to chamomile have occurred. Allergies are more likely if you are allergic to members of the daisy family.

Rosemary (*Rosmarinus officinalis*)

The essential oil of rosemary is used in many skin care products. Research indicates the oil can help kill bacteria and fight skin inflammation. Minor bacterial or fungal infections of the skin are commonly treated with creams or ointments containing rosemary. The antimicrobial properties of rosemary are useful for allergic skin conditions, such as eczema, that are frequently complicated by bacterial skin infections. *Typical dosage*: Follow manufacturer's directions. *Caution*: Topical rosemary essential oil can cause a rash with sun exposure; discontinue use if this occurs.

Chapter 10
Herbal Remedies

CR&O

Humans have relied on plants for thousands of years as natural sources of medicines. We know many of these plants contain amazing therapeutic substances in rich array. In fact, several drugs on the market were originally isolated from plants and then synthesized. Yet we have only just begun to identify and classify many of these plant substances.

As scientific knowledge of the health effects of botanicals has grown, so has consumer awareness. Greater numbers of people are again purchasing herbs for self care. Having withstood the test of time in cultures around the world, medicinal herbs are a popular choice for those who seek treatments that are effective but gentle with fewer side effects than drugs.

But some caution is warranted: Herbs and dietary supplements are not regulated nearly as closely as drugs in the U.S. Some products are tainted with contaminants or toxins, or do not contain the amounts of ingredients printed on the label. To find quality products, carefully research each herb before you buy and only purchase products made by reputable companies. The online resource ConsumerLab.com conducts independent research on a selection of herbal products and other dietary supplements and publishes the results. Physicians trained in integrative medicine can also give you advice about herbs. For a glossary of herbal and botanical terms, turn to Appendix G.

Besides effectiveness and quality, potential interactions between drugs and herbs are another area of concern. Your best defense is to keep your physician and pharmacist informed about all of the supplements and drugs you are taking so they can help you guard against drug interactions and side effects.

Adverse effects from herbs and supplements may pose a particular risk for certain groups of people. Pregnant or nursing women, children, and people with kidney or liver disease or other chronic disorders are especially vulnerable. People at risk for harm should only take herbal therapies under the supervision of a physician.

Herbs for Allergy Relief

Herbs have long been a mainstay for allergic ailments like hay fever and asthma. Certain botanicals are known to have anti-inflammatory and allergy-fighting effects. These herbs work to decrease the body's production of chemicals that incite inflammation and allergies. Other therapeutic plants have specific actions as natural antihistamines.

But herbs possess an antihistamine activity that is distinctly different from that of drugs. The substance histamine is produced and released by specialized cells in your immune system called mast cells. These cells release stored histamine in response to pollens or other allergy-causing substances. The released histamine then triggers allergy symptoms such as sneezing, wheezing or watery eyes. In this chemical cascade of events, antihistamine drugs stop histamine after it is released by blocking the histamine receptors located on the surface of body cells. Herbs with

Elizabeth Smoots MD

natural antihistamine activity, however, act by preventing the formation of histamine in the first place. They're often referred to as mast-cell stabilizers since the herbs calm down your body's mast cells, making the cells less likely to produce and release stored supplies of histamine.

This stabilizing process takes time. Many herbs that provide allergy relief are slow to start acting, with symptom improvements coming in two to four weeks. So don't wait until your allergy symptoms have already gotten out of hand. Start taking herbal remedies at least two weeks before allergy season strikes for best results.

Butterbur (*Petasites hybridus*)

Best known for migraine prevention, butterbur is one of the primary herbs in my armamentarium against hay fever and asthma. The herb boasts notable anti-inflammatory and anti-allergy effects. As a natural antihistamine, it stabilizes mast cells and prevents the release of histamine. It also inhibits your body's production of the inflammatory substance leukotriene in response to allergies. The evidence for a beneficial effect from butterbur is backed up by substantial research. In fact, allergy studies show the effectiveness of butterbur is equal to antihistamine drugs like fexofenadine or cetirizine but with fewer side effects. *Typical dosage*: 25 to 50 milligrams two to three times a day of a standardized extract that has been processed to remove pyrrolizidine alkaloids. *Caution:* Butterbur naturally contains pyrrolizidine alkaloids that may damage your liver. Only use extracts that are completely free of these potentially dangerous chemicals. The herb should be avoided by pregnant or nursing women, young children, and people with kidney or liver disease. Those who are allergic to daisies could also react to butterbur.

Chinese Skullcap (*Scutellaria baicalensis*)

The nickname for Scutellaria is "scute." Practitioners of traditional Chinese medicine have long utilized the herb to treat allergies such as allergic rhinitis, asthma and eczema. Scute reduces responsiveness to allergies by stabilizing mast cells. It also inhibits the body's production of inflammatory substances like leukotrienes in response to allergies. In addition, scute acts as a calming agent to reduce anxiety and stress, and offers broad-spectrum activity against viruses and bacteria. *Typical dosage*: 3 to 9 grams per day as part of a combination herbal tincture. *Caution:* Liver injury has been reported with skullcap products, though the adverse effect may have been caused by contamination with the herb germander. Drug interactions are known to occur.

Albizzia (*Albizzia lebbeck*)

A member of the legume family, this plant grows into a large tree nicknamed "rattle-pod." Ayurvedic medicine in India has traditionally employed the dried stem bark to treat allergic rhinitis, asthma and eczema. The herb has anti-inflammatory and anti-allergic properties. It works as a natural antihistamine to prevent the release of histamine from mast cells. *Typical dosage*: 1.5 to 3.0 grams per day as part of a combination herbal formula or tincture.

Boswellia (*Boswellia serrata*)

The gummy tree resin is a popular herbal remedy for asthma in India. Boswellia is also known as Indian Frankincense. It's a potent inhibitor of leukotrienes and other inflammatory substances that aggravate wheezing and coughing in asthma. Several studies have shown improved breathing measurements and a reduced need for drug therapy in asthmatics taking boswellia. It is especially useful in people

Elizabeth Smoots MD

who have both asthma and gastrointestinal problems such as gastritis or inflammatory bowel disease. *Typical dosage*: 300 to 400 milligrams three times a day of a standardized extract containing 37.5 percent boswellic acid. *Caution*: The herb's safety has not been established in children, pregnant or nursing women, or people with liver or kidney disease.

Stinging Nettle (*Urtica dioica*)

The name of this nettle comes from the fine hairs on its leaves and stems that inflict persistent burning pain. Research shows all of the above-ground parts of this tall green plant have medicinal value. The herb possesses anti-inflammatory and mast-cell-stabilizing effects that are used to treat allergies and allergic rhinitis, or hay fever. Research results are very limited. *Typical dosage:* 300 milligrams two to three times a day of freeze-dried nettle leaf as needed to control allergy symptoms. *Caution*: Nettle has the potential to interact with several medications, including those for high blood pressure, diabetes, anxiety and insomnia.

Tylophora (*Tylophora asthmatica*)

Tylophora is a climbing perennial plant that grows in India. The leaves have long been utilized as a treatment for asthma. Indian practitioners of ayurvedic medicine also avail themselves of the herb for respiratory conditions such as allergic rhinitis, bronchitis and the common cold. Studies have only been done on its use in asthma. *Typical dosage:* 200 milligrams two times a day of the dried leaves as a crude bulk herb or capsule. *Caution*: Little research has been conducted about safety, so the herb should not be used by children, pregnant or nursing women, or people with kidney or liver disease.

Tinospora (*Tinospora cordifolia*)

Some evidence shows that whole plant extracts of tinospora may significantly decrease sneezing and nasal congestion in people with allergic rhinitis. The herb is thought to work by inhibiting the release of histamine from mast cells. *Typical dosage:* Amounts of specific extracts vary by brand. *Caution:* Little research has been conducted about safety, so the herb should not be used by children, pregnant or nursing women, or people with kidney or liver disease.

Feverfew (*Tanacetum parthenium*)

Commonly taken to prevent migraine headaches, feverfew possesses anti-inflammatory activity that may ease hay fever symptoms. However, this has not been confirmed in studies. *Typical dosage:* 50 milligrams once or twice daily of powdered, freeze-dried feverfew leaves, most often standardized to 0.2 to 0.35 percent parthenolide. *Caution:* Use of the herb, especially chewing the fresh leaves, may cause mouth ulcers or lip swelling; discontinue the product if this occurs. If you are allergic to daisies, be aware that feverfew belongs to the same family. The herb has blood-thinning activity and should not be combined with blood-thinning drugs or taken before surgery. Do not take during pregnancy.

Herbs to Aid Respiratory Tract

Several common herbs can sooth your airways and help thin and liquefy mucus and expel it from your body. These nonspecific actions help calm down allergies and support the health of the nasal passages and airways as well as your entire respiratory system.

Ginger (*Zingiber officinale*)

The underground stem, or rhizome, of this plant is one of my go-to herbs for allergies and other respiratory conditions. It can break up and thin mucus as well as reduce mucus production. I have found that ginger's anti-inflammatory action can help relieve allergies, sinus infections, sore throats, coughs and colds. *Typical dosage:* To make ginger tea, combine 2 cups of water with an inch of fresh ginger rhizome chopped into small pieces. Bring the mixture to a boil in a saucepan, then reduce the heat and simmer for 15 to 20 minutes. Strain and serve warm. Drink a cup one to three times per day. *Caution:* While ginger is usually used to treat nausea and indigestion, large amounts of the herb can create heartburn and nausea in some people. Ginger has blood-thinning activity and should not be combined with blood-thinning drugs or taken before surgery.

Garlic (*Allium sativum*)

The pungent bulb has anti-inflammatory properties that can help calm down allergic rhinitis, or hay fever. Garlic also acts as an antibacterial and antiviral agent to help prevent upper respiratory infections and sinusitis. *Typical dosage*: Garlic powder extract standardized to provide 4 to 8 milligrams of allicin daily; or chew 1 to 2 fresh garlic cloves a day. *Caution:* Garlic has blood-thinning activity and should not be combined with blood-thinning drugs or taken before surgery.

Licorice (*Glycyrrhiza glabra*)

A revered remedy throughout herbal folklore, licorice has traditionally been used to relieve sore throats and coughs. The potent properties of its underground stems, or rhizomes, include soothing irritated mucous membranes, calming inflamed airways, and breaking up accumulations of mucus.

Licorice has a cortisol-sparing effect that may assist people in tapering down on cortisone medications. The herb is commonly employed as a harmonizing agent in herbal formulas for allergies, asthma, upper respiratory infections, and a host of other maladies. *Typical dosage:* As a treatment for sore throat, suck on licorice lozenges several times daily for a few days. Take no more than 500 milligrams a day of the crude root for short-term use (less than two weeks) without your physician's supervision. For longer-term use, take even less (no more than 300 milligrams a day) and have your response monitored by your physician. *Caution:* The active ingredient glycyrrhizin in licorice can cause high blood pressure, salt and water retention, low blood potassium, heartbeat irregularities, or kidney failure. Do not take the herb at all, except with the close supervision of a qualified physician, if you have heart or kidney disease or if you use blood pressure medications or blood thinners. Licorice is not advised for pregnant or nursing women.

Thyme (*Thymus vulgaris*)

The culinary herb thyme provides an effective remedy for colds, coughs and upper respiratory infections. Thymol, a substance in the herb's aromatic essential oil, is the chief active ingredient. The herb helps ease coughing, relieves congestion, reduces inflammation, and generally supports the body in fighting viral infections. It can also help thin and expel phlegm in children and adults with copious mucus production related to colds, bronchitis, sinusitis, allergies or asthma. *Typical dosage:* To make thyme tea, steep one to two teaspoons of fresh or dried thyme in one cup of water. Strain and drink warm several times a day.

To make thyme syrup, pour one cup of boiling water over 1 to 2 tablespoons of dried thyme, or 4 tablespoons of fresh thyme. Steep for 15 minutes. Strain out the leaves and add 1/4 cup of honey and 1 teaspoon of lemon juice to the remaining liquid. Take 1 to 2 tablespoons of thyme syrup every two to four hours as needed. Do not give honey to infants under age 12 months since it can cause infant botulism. The syrup keeps in the refrigerator for up to one week.

Peppermint (*Mentha piperita*)

This familiar herb has anti-inflammatory properties that may be beneficial for relieving coughs, colds and allergies. Peppermint can help loosen phlegm, thin mucus, and decongest a stuffy nose. *Typical dosage:* To make peppermint tea, combine 1 teaspoon of the dried herb with 1 cup of boiling water and let steep for 15 minutes. Strain and serve warm. You can repeat the process two to three times a day. Throat lozenges are also available; look for those with 5 to 10 milligrams of menthol. *Caution:* Do not give products with menthol to young children under the age of three years. At all ages, peppermint may worsen symptoms of heartburn or esophageal reflux.

Herbs for Immune Support

Some herbs promote normal functioning of your immune system and help it resist disease. These so-called "adaptogenic herbs" increase your body's ability to adjust to the demands of physical, chemical and biological stress. They also improve the general health of your immune system and make it less reactive to situations and substances that trigger allergies.

Astragalus (*Astragalus membranaceus*)

The root of this plant is used to strengthen and regulate the immune system. It is often taken during cold and flu season to ward off upper respiratory tract infections, especially among people who suffer from frequent colds. *Typical dosage:* Capsules with 1 to 3 grams a day of the dried, powdered root. To make tea, bring 2 to 4 cups of water to a boil and add 3 to 6 tablespoons of dried, chopped astragalus root. Steep for 15 minutes and serve warm a couple of times a day. You can also cook with the fresh root, simmering it in herb-flavored soups; be sure to discard the root before serving. *Caution:* Do not use astragalus to remedy an acute respiratory infection; it is traditionally used in Chinese medicine as a preventive agent. If you suffer from an autoimmune disorder, take astragalus only under a physician's supervision.

Ashwagandha (*Withania somnifera*)

Known for its calming and quieting effects, ashwagandha is popularly used to soothe anxiety and tension and improve sleep. The herb can help turn off a racing mind; this quality is especially beneficial when repetitive thoughts keep you awake or prevent you from falling back to sleep. In addition, ashwagandha can help strengthen and support your immune system and your lungs. *Typical dosage:* 500 milligrams two to three times a day of a standardized extract containing 2 to 5 percent withanolides; or 0.5 to 2 grams two to three times daily of the crude herb as dried root powder. *Caution:* Do not take with sedative drugs.

Rhodiola (*Rhodiola rosea*)

The Scandinavians prize this herb, also called "arctic root," for its ability to increase energy and improve mood. It is also used to alleviate mild depression. Rhodiola works as an adaptogen to reduce the frequency of colds and respiratory infections during dark winter months. This action is especially helpful for people with allergies who tend to get sinus infections or bronchitis. *Typical dosage:* 100 to 250 milligrams once or twice a day of a standardized extract containing 3 to 5 percent rosavin and 0.8 to 1.0 percent salidroside. Start with a low dose and gradually increase to the upper typical amount as needed.

Reishi (*Ganoderma lucidum*)

An edible tree fungus, reishi is frequently used in China to alleviate asthma and other allergic conditions. The traditional healing herb is thought to help normalize immune function. Reishi also possesses anti-viral and anti-cancer properties. *Typical dosage:* 2 to 6 grams per day of the crude dried mushroom taken with meals, or an equivalent amount of an extract. *Caution:* Reishi has blood-thinning activity and should not be combined with blood-thinning drugs or taken before surgery.

Chapter 11
Dietary Supplements

ভ্ঠ

Interest in unconventional approaches to health care has grown in recent years. More than two out of five adults in the U.S. say they use complementary and alternative therapies to treat their health problems. Among people with allergy symptoms, the proportion is even higher. An estimated 60 percent of allergy sufferers try a natural product at some point. Supplements of vitamins, minerals, essential oils, and other dietary components are among the most popular of these products.

But caution is warranted in buying dietary supplements, just like it is for purchasing herbal remedies. Both types of products are not regulated nearly as closely as drugs in the U.S. Some supplements are tainted with contaminants or toxins, or do not contain ingredients in the amounts claimed on the label.

Carefully research each supplement you want to buy and only purchase products made by reputable companies. ConsumerLab.com conducts independent research on herbs and dietary supplements and publishes the results online. Physicians trained in integrative medicine are also a good source of advice.

Potential interactions between dietary supplements and drugs are another important issue. Regularly provide your physician and pharmacist with an updated list of all of the supplements and drugs you are taking. Giving them access to the most complete information enables them to help you watch for drug interactions and side effects.

Certain groups of people are at particular risk for adverse effects from dietary supplements. Especially vulnerable are pregnant or nursing women, children, and people with kidney or liver disease or other chronic disorders. People at risk for harm should not take dietary supplements except under the supervision of a physician.

Principal Supplements

Fish Oil

The omega-3 fatty acids contained in fish oil are essential for good health. You must get the fats from your diet since your body cannot make them. But most people are deficient since they eat little fish or other dietary sources. You may further compound a deficiency when you consume a lot of processed foods and vegetable oils containing omega-6 fats. An excellent way to restore a healthier balance of dietary fats is to eat more fish or take fish oil supplements.

Fish oil supplements typically contain large quantities of omega-3 fatty acids. In sufficient amounts the fats have anti-inflammatory effects on your entire body. Reducing underlying inflammation helps your body break up mucous plugs and swelling to relieve allergy symptoms. Research indicates that daily supplementation with fish oil can also help alleviate exercise-induced asthma and improve eczema. *Typical dosage*: Look on the label for the amounts of the two main kinds of omega-3 fats, docosahexaenoic acid (DHA) and eicosapentaenoic acid (EPA). The EPA component of fish oil is especially beneficial for allergies. For mild allergies, a daily dose of 500 to 600 milligrams of EPA and 200 to 400 milligrams of DHA may be sufficient for general health. If you have more severe allergies or asthma, aim for 1,000 to 1,200 milligrams of EPA and 400 to 800 milligrams of DHA per day in your supplement. Take it with a meal containing fat for the best absorption. Fish oil comes in capsules or liquid concentrate; look for molecularly distilled products. Vegan sources of omega-3 fats derived from algae are also available. *Caution*: Do not take more than 1,200 milligrams a day of either EPA or DHA without the advice of your health care provider. Since fish oil has blood-thinning activity, it should not be combined with blood-thinning drugs or taken before surgery.

Probiotics

Probiotics are natural food ingredients containing live microorganisms that have beneficial health effects. A variety of different bacteria and yeasts have long been used to create probiotics by people around the globe. Common examples of these cultured or fermented foods include yogurt, buttermilk, sour cream, kefir, tempeh, miso and raw sauerkraut. I am a big fan of eating probiotic foods. Consuming them frequently helps replenish the friendly bacteria in the digestive tract. The good bacteria can improve your digestion, protect your intestinal lining, and help keep your immune system functioning well. Some studies indicate that probiotic foods or supplements may help ease asthma, eczema and other allergic disorders. Typical dosage: 3 to 10 billion colony-forming units per day as a capsule or liquid concentrate, or six ounces of yogurt. You can further boost the activity of helpful gut bacteria by slowly increasing your intake of soluble fiber;

good sources include fruits, vegetables, beans, flaxseeds, oats and barley. Caution: Consult a physician before giving probiotics to infants, the elderly, or people with chronic disorders or weak immune systems.

Quercetin

It's a bioflavonoid found just under the skin of citrus, berries, apples, tomatoes, onions, garlic, kale, broccoli and green beans. Red wine and tea are also good sources. Quercetin has antioxidant, anti-inflammatory and anti-allergy properties. It works as a natural antihistamine to prevent the release of histamine from your body's mast cells. These properties are more pronounced when you take the supplements in advance of an allergy exposure or use them continuously during allergy season. *Typical dosage*: 200 to 400 milligrams two to three times per day. *Caution*: Do not take during pregnancy.

Vitamin C

Often suggested as a remedy for allergies, vitamin C, also known as ascorbic acid, may have an anti-allergy effect. Several small studies show benefit, while other research does not. One small study found that a dose of 1,500 milligrams of vitamin C, taken all at once before exercise, helped improve exercise-induced asthma. *Typical dosage*: 500 to 2,000 milligrams per day in divided doses. Alternatively, eat plenty of foods rich in vitamin C such as citrus, melons, berries, broccoli and bell peppers. *Caution*: The tolerable upper intake for vitamin C is 2,000 milligrams a day for adults; doses above this limit are more likely to cause adverse effects. Larger amounts may cause nausea, diarrhea, or an increased risk of kidney stones. Drug interactions are known to occur.

Vitamin D

A deficiency of vitamin D impairs the normal immune function of your body. Low levels can aggravate allergic conditions and increase your susceptibility to upper respiratory infections. Allergy sufferers who frequently contract sinus infections or colds are especially at risk. Vitamin D-3, or cholecalciferol, is the most effective type of supplement. *Typical dosage*: The Institute of Medicine recommends 600 international units of vitamin D a day for ages one year to 70 years. After that, the dose goes up to 800 international units per day. These are general recommendations for the U.S. population as a whole. Many people need larger amounts than this, so consult with your physician for personalized advice, and ask if you need a vitamin D blood test. *Caution*: The Institute of Medicine has set the tolerable upper limit for vitamin D supplements at 4,000 international units per day for adults and children age nine years and older; amounts under this limit are unlikely to cause adverse health effects. To minimize your risk of toxicity, don't exceed this amount without your physician's approval. Excess amounts can cause high blood levels of calcium, kidney problems, and calcium deposits in your body's tissues.

Other Supplements

Magnesium

Levels of this mineral are often low in people with asthma. Magnesium is sometimes given intravenously in emergency rooms to treat asthma attacks. Several studies show that asthmatics who regularly take the mineral by mouth have stronger breathing muscles and fewer severe symptoms. *Typical dosage*: 400 milligrams orally once a day. *Caution*: Magnesium can cause diarrhea. The glycinate form of the mineral produces less of a laxative effect than do the citrate or oxide forms.

Selenium

Selenium is a trace mineral that has antioxidant and anti-inflammatory properties. It helps protect your cell membranes from oxidative damage caused by free radicals. A deficiency of selenium may play a role in flare ups of asthma and the development of asthma early in life. Some evidence indicates supplementing with selenium may be beneficial for people with asthma. *Typical dosage*: 200 micrograms per day. *Caution*: Excess amounts of selenium can cause hair loss, depression, nervousness, nausea and vomiting.

Coenzyme Q10

CoQ10, or ubiquinone, is a potent antioxidant that occurs naturally in your body's cells. Levels of the substance often drop too low in people with asthma. Preliminary evidence suggests that CoQ10 supplements may be beneficial for some people who suffer from asthma. *Typical dosage*: 100 milligrams once or twice a day. Oil-based soft gels may be better absorbed than dry powder tablets or capsules. *Caution*: People with heart disease or other chronic conditions should only take CoQ10 under a doctor's direction.

Bromelain

Encompassing several different protein-digesting enzymes derived from pineapple, bromelain may help regulate and support your immune system and reduce inflammation. Several studies have found that bromelain supplements may provide some benefit for people with sinus infections. The facial cavities around the nose get infected all too often in many allergy sufferers. *Typical dosage*: The amount of supplement varies by brand. Alternatively, you can simply enjoy consuming more fresh pineapple in your diet. *Caution*: Bromelain has blood-thinning activity and should not be combined with blood-thinning drugs or taken before surgery. It should also not be used by anyone allergic to pineapple.

Bee Pollen

Some people claim that consuming local bee pollen can improve hay fever. But there is no significant scientific evidence to date that it is effective. *Typical dosage*: It's usually started in miniscule amounts and then gradually increased. *Caution*: Serious allergic reactions and anaphylaxis have occurred, so use bee pollen only under the supervision of a physician.

Honey

A natural sweetener containing trace amounts of nutrients, honey has traditionally been used to treat wounds as well as coughs and hay fever. For people with allergies, consumption of raw, local honey is commonly touted as a natural way to build immunity to the pollens in an area. However, the one published study that looked at honey and hay fever failed to find any benefit. *Typical dosage*: One to two tablespoons one or more times per day. *Caution*: Do not give honey to infants less than 12 months old since it can cause infant botulism.

Chapter 12
Mind-Body Therapies

ᘓᘔᗥᘐ

The intimate association between your mind and body plays an important role in allergic conditions. When considering hay fever, asthma, eczema or other allergies, we do not need to look far to find convincing evidence of a mind-body connection.

Take the example of a severe allergy to cats. Just looking at a picture of a cat can trigger sneezing and watery eyes in some highly allergic individuals. In this situation, even though there's no real cat around, the body still reacts strongly to the idea of "Uh-oh. There's a cat." The physical symptoms produced in response to feelings and thoughts are a representation of the mind's learned way of dealing with the allergies.

Emotional stress of all kinds can also trigger allergic reactions. Symptoms of asthma or hay fever may ignite when problems heat up at work, school or home. Likewise, moving to a new location, death in the family, or the breakup of an important relationship can precipitate an asthma attack or touch off a flare of allergies.

Fortunately, you can take advantage of the very same mind-body connection to calm distressing health conditions. A number of relaxation techniques can help you change your mental and emotional state which, in turn, influences the symptoms of asthma or allergies that you experience.

The key is to find a relaxation technique that you are willing to do regularly. Practicing the exercises on a daily basis, or at least a couple of times a week, provides much greater benefit than doing them sporadically. With regular practice your brain changes its electrical pattern of firing. Research shows that individual nerve cells as well as entire areas of your brain actually change their physical structure when you follow a routine of mind-body exercises.

Look over the popular techniques below and choose one or more that you are interested in trying. After you get started with the basics, you can continue to improve your techniques with further reading, audio and video recordings, classes, or private instruction.

Journaling

Writing down your thoughts and feelings is a simple way to allow your mind to influence your body. You can use a notebook, a journal, or a diary to record what's going on with your life and how you feel about it. Also chart your symptoms and any factors that may have triggered your allergies. Other useful items to record include the timing of your medications or treatments, your activities, your emotional state, and your overall stress level.

Scheduling a time to write in your journal every day can be very therapeutic for hay fever, eczema, asthma and many other health conditions. It provides an emotional release to help you manage and relieve stress. Your factual observations can also provide valuable clues about possible underlying causes of your allergic disorder.

Elizabeth Smoots MD

Breathwork

Learning to influence your breath can have many health benefits. Scientific studies show simple breathing exercises may help increase energy, calm frazzled nerves, and enhance immune functioning. This can result in improved digestion, circulation, blood pressure and pulse as well as fewer problems with chronic conditions such as allergies. In fact, breathwork is the simplest and most effective relaxation technique I know for bringing greater harmony to your whole self, including your mind, body and spirit.

Try the following basic breathing exercises for a few minutes twice a day while sitting in a quiet place.

Yogic Tongue Position

Touch the tip of your tongue to the back of your upper front teeth. Then slide it up just a bit, until it is lightly touching the ridge of hard tissue between the teeth and the palate. Maintain this tongue position throughout all the breathing exercises.

Breathing Deeply

These techniques will help you take deeper breaths. The first technique is called "belly breathing." Place one hand on your stomach. Take a deep breath and feel your stomach expand. Hold for a few seconds, then slowly exhale. The second technique is to exhale first. At the beginning of each breathing exercise, begin with an out breath followed by an in breath and so forth.

Bellows Breath

This exercise helps raise energy and increase alertness. Rapidly breathe in and out through your nose, keeping your mouth lightly closed. Practice the exercise for 15 seconds initially. You can then gradually increase the length of time.

Slow, Quiet, Deep

To reduce anger or anxiety, try making your breaths slower, deeper, quieter, and more regular.

4-7-8 breath

Also known as the "relaxing breath," the 4-7-8 breath is an especially powerful stress-control technique. Inhale quietly through your nose to the count of four. Hold your breath to the count of seven. Then exhale noisily through your mouth to the count of eight. Do four breath cycles at a time, twice a day. After you practice for a month or two, you can increase to eight breath cycles at each sitting.

Breathwork Resources

For additional information and breathing practice, I recommend listening to the audio recording *Breathing: The Master Key to Self Healing* by Andrew Weil, MD.

Progressive Muscle Relaxation

The technique involves tensing and relaxing muscle groups throughout your body in an orderly sequence. Typically, each muscle is tensed for 8 to 10 seconds, and then relaxed to let the tension go. The process is repeated in different muscles in a progressive fashion, starting at your toes and working up to your head, or vice versa. Progressively contracting and then relaxing your muscles helps to release both physical and mental tension, according to research.

Guided Imagery

Imagery is what you see in your mind's eye. Research shows the same parts of the brain activate when you imagine something as when you actually experience it. These changes in brain activity can alter your heart rate, blood pressure, hormone levels and immune function. So, visually thinking about something actually changes the physiology of your body.

The most effective guided imagery does not limit itself solely to the sense of sight. Incorporating your other senses, such as smell, taste, hearing and touch, works even more effectively to evoke emotions and enhance the benefits you gain from guided imagery.

HEALTH TIP FROM DR. SMOOTS

Guided Imagery Resources

A large number of audio recordings are available on the market to help you get started learning about guided imagery. The recordings usually lead you step by step through a guided imagery sequence. A good place to begin is with the many first-rate audio recordings by Belleruth Naparstek at *www.healthjourneys.com*.

Meditation

Numerous studies have demonstrated the health benefits of meditation. The term means directed concentration. People who meditate learn to focus their attention on the breath, repeated words or phrases, or a sound, body sensation or visual image.

In the process they elicit the relaxation response. Heart rate and breathing slow. Blood pressure and levels of the stress hormone cortisol decrease.

Scientists have found that meditation is an effective antidote for anger and worry. It's also beneficial for dealing with chronic pain, panic disorder, anxiety, depression, high blood pressure, heart disease, asthma, cancer, irritable bowel, psoriasis and many other ailments.

You can learn more about the ancient mind-body practice in several ways. A wide variety of books, tapes, seminars and classes provide instruction on how to do meditation. Physicians trained in integrative medicine can also help you get started.

To begin with, here are some simple meditation tips:

- Pick a place and time free of distractions, for example, on arising in the morning.
- Sit on a comfortable chair or cushion with your spine erect.
- Close your eyes and quietly take slow, deep breaths.
- Turn your attention to a specific focus. You can concentrate on your breath or repeated words, phrases, sounds or visual images. Each time your mind wanders gently bring it back to your focus.
- Learn creative ways to meditate 10 to 20 minutes each day. You can practice it while falling asleep, eating, or doing routine chores or activities in a safe place.

Meditation Resources

I suggest reading *Meditation for Beginners* by Jack Kornfield and *Wherever You Go, There You Are* by Jon Kabat-Zinn. You will find audio recordings for guided meditation practice by the same authors as well as other similar authors at *www.soundstrue.com*.

Hypnotherapy

Hypnosis involves inducing a trance-like state of inward concentration and focused attention. The unconscious mind becomes more open to ideas and suggestions in the hypnotic state. You may receive treatments from a trained hypnotherapist, or you can learn to do self-hypnosis yourself. Either way, positive ideas, suggestions and images can be used in such a way that they are helpful to you for improving your mental and physical health.

Here's an example of how hypnosis works. If you have asthma, for example, you can imagine air easily moving through your breathing tubes during inspiration and expiration. Your unconscious mind then sends these thoughts as nerve impulses throughout your body. This can affect your airways and your lungs as well as other organs and tissues. It also influences your production of hormones and the function of your nervous system and immune system in ways that are not possible in ordinary states of consciousness.

Research has shown that hypnosis can benefit hay fever and asthma. The technique may alleviate or prevent allergic reactions and restore balance to your immune system. Once your immune system has quieted down, it can learn less harmful ways of responding to allergy-causing substances.

The results can make a significant difference. Patients with hay fever may experience allergic flares less often after receiving hypnotherapy. Likewise, asthma patients treated with hypnosis have been shown to have fewer asthma attacks, better breathing function, and reduced reliance on drugs in some studies.

Hypnosis Resources

For audio recordings about medical hypnosis and self-hypnosis, I recommend those made by Steven Gurgevich, PhD. You can get more information about the recordings at *www.healingwithhypnosis.com* and *www.soundstrue.com*.

Biofeedback

Biofeedback involves using signals from your own body to improve your health. The technique allows you to alter the temperature of your skin or the tension in your muscles, for example. You can also learn to influence your brain activity, blood pressure, heart rate and other bodily functions that normally are not controlled voluntarily.

The set up usually involves a computer and way to connect your body to the computer such as a transducer or set of electrodes. The computer translates the electrical signals from the electrodes into an image on your computer screen. During the biofeedback process, you learn how to change a particular bodily process in such a way that it causes the computer to bring the pictured monitor image into the desired target range.

Physicians are currently using biofeedback to treat a growing list of health conditions. These include asthma and other allergic conditions as well as heart disease, movement disorders, anxiety and pain. A good place to start, if you're interested in learning more about biofeedback, is to get a consultation with your physician.

Chapter 13
Manual Medicine

CR&O

From birth until death, all of us have a basic need to be touched. With the advent of technology, however, the art of the so-called "laying on of hands" has largely been lost in modern medicine. Bodywork, or manual therapy, has been developed in part to help fill this void.

In manual medicine, the practitioner's hands are seen as tools that are used to diagnose and treat health conditions. Specialized techniques are used to massage, manipulate, stretch, apply pressure, or therapeutically touch the body. The techniques are employed to treat a wide range of physical disorders. Emotions that are stored in the muscles, skeleton and other tissues may also find release with manual therapies.

If you are interested in a treatment involving manual medicine, consult your physician to learn about the potential benefits for your health condition. Asking for a referral is a good way to locate qualified practitioners in your area.

Osteopathic Treatment

Manual therapies play an important role in the system of medicine called osteopathy. According to osteopathic principles, manipulation of your muscles and bones may help restore normal structure and improve blood flow to an injured area.

Therapeutic changes in your musculoskeletal system may also have healing effects on disorders in corresponding organs or tissues of your body. For example, osteopathic techniques like rib-raising can help treat asthma or lower respiratory infections such as bronchitis or pneumonia.

To alleviate hay fever, treatments to improve the structural mechanics of the bones of your skull, neck and chest can increase your body's ability to withstand allergy-causing agents. The osteopathic treatments serve to normalize your nerve function, improve your circulation, and increase drainage. Bringing balance to allergy-related areas of your body is seen as clearing the way so hay fever symptoms can improve.

Craniosacral Therapy

Originating in the field of osteopathic medicine, a treatment called craniosacral therapy has gained widespread popularity and acceptance in many other health professions. Medical doctors, naturopaths, chiropractors, and massage therapists are among the practitioners who regularly perform the techniques of craniosacral therapy.

The modality uses gentle touch to manipulate the bones of your skull as well as your lower spine and pelvis. The technique is thought to normalize the flow of cerebrospinal fluid that surrounds and protects your central nervous system. The goal is to restore the optimal rhythm, or wave, of fluid movement in order to improve health.

Craniosacral therapy is used to treat a number of health conditions. In people with allergic disorders, craniosacral therapy can help improve sinus drainage and relieve congestion in the nasal passages and other areas of the respiratory system.

Massage Therapy

Many of us lose flexibility and develop muscle knots and bands of tension with age or disability. Massage therapy is designed to help open and lengthen your body and release muscle tightness. It does this with a variety of hands-on techniques such as rubbing, stroking, stretching, kneading, lifting, rolling, shaking, tapping, vibrating, holding and applying pressure.

Research has shown that massage may be beneficial for conditions with a strong mind-body connection such as asthma and allergic disorders. A large body of evidence indicates the technique can help alleviate stress, pain, anxiety, insomnia and chronic fatigue. It may also increase soft tissue suppleness, stimulate circulation, and improve your overall sense of well-being.

Massage therapists often specialize in treating certain groups of people such as injured athletes, infants, seniors, abuse survivors or disabled patients. Look for therapists who have experience with groups of people similar to you, and who have met the requirements for licensing and credentialing in your state. Massage is generally not advised if you have an infectious skin disease.

Chapter 14
Whole Medical Systems

CR&O

Complete systems of medical theory and practice have evolved over time in different cultures around the world. Those that have developed apart from conventional, or Western, medicine are sometimes called whole medical systems. Traditional Chinese Medicine and Ayurveda are well recognized and respected as major traditions in the East. Whole systems in the West include homeopathy and naturopathy as well as Native American and South American medicine.

Many of these systems share the belief that the body has the power to heal itself. They often incorporate ideas and techniques that involve the patient's mind, body and spirit in their healing practices. Each whole medical system has its own diagnostic and treatment approaches that can be employed to bring relief for allergy sufferers.

Traditional Chinese Medicine

Originating in China more than 2,000 years ago, traditional Chinese medicine sees the human body in terms of the flow of energy and the harmony between opposing forces. Disease is created when the forces get out of balance or energy flow becomes restricted. To find health and harmony, the opposing forces of yin and yang must be brought back into balance. Likewise, the body's energy, qi, must flow freely without restrictions or blockages to avoid illness. Treatments in traditional Chinese medicine may involve diet, exercise, lifestyle changes, acupuncture and herbs and are usually highly individualized.

Herbal Remedies

Traditional Chinese medicine is known for its use of formulas that contain a large number of herbal ingredients. Several studies have shown significant improvements in the symptoms of allergic rhinitis, asthma and eczema among people treated with Chinese herbal formulas. *Caution:* Some Chinese herb formulations have been adulterated with toxins or unlisted ingredients. It is imperative to work only with fully licensed and credentialed practitioners of traditional Chinese medicine. Check with your state medical board or other appropriate licensing agency to find out what requirements have been established in your state.

Diet and Exercise

Traditional Chinese medicine advises patients with allergies or asthma to avoid dampness and phlegm-producing foods. It is especially important to limit raw or cold foods, dairy products and peanut butter, according to the discipline. Protect your neck with a scarf or coat against the cold, especially on wet or windy days. Build vitality by doing regular exercise such as qigong or tai chi. In addition, practice a relaxation technique such as visualizing the movement of energy, or qi, throughout your body.

Elizabeth Smoots MD

Acupuncture

The placement of acupuncture needles at points along lines called meridians is often a component of Chinese medical treatment. Practitioners frequently treat acute asthma attacks with acupuncture. They may also combine acupuncture with herbal medicine in the treatment of asthma and allergic diseases. Acupuncture is often provided as a complement to conventional medicine in a comprehensive treatment plan designed for asthma. *Caution*: Check with your state medical board for the requirements of acupuncture licensure in your state.

Ayurveda

Founded 5,000 years ago in India, Ayurveda means "life knowledge." The holistic discipline emphasizes the interconnectedness of your mind, body and spirit. All must be in balance to attain health and happiness, according to the philosophy.

People are characterized as having one or more mind-body types in Ayurveda. Distinctive attributes are associated with each type, also known as constitutions or energies of nature. The first type is vata, which illustrates the principles of movement and change. People with a predominantly vata constitution have a thin body type and are creative and lively. They are prone to suffer from anxiety, insomnia and irregular digestion. The second type, pitta, is characterized by the digestion of food and ideas. Those with an abundance of pitta in their nature tend to be muscular and intelligent. But they can easily become angry or jealous. The third type is kapha, which stands for the principle of stability. People with considerable kapha in their constitution often have a heavy frame and calm, stable moods. They are prone to obesity and diabetes, and are often resistant to healthy lifestyle change.

Disease occurs when all aspects of a person's constitution are not in proper balance. Ayurveda incorporates nutrition, culinary spices, herbal therapies, yoga, massage, meditation, fasting and other cleansing methods to restore healthful harmony to the person. The techniques used for the prevention and treatment of disease are often complex and very individualized.

Scientific studies have been performed on ayurvedic herbal formulas and healing practices. Preliminary results have shown improvements in immune function and allergy symptoms in people with asthma or hay fever. *Caution:* Some ayurvedic herbal formulations have been adulterated with toxins or unlisted ingredients. It is imperative to work only with fully licensed and credentialed practitioners of ayurvedic medicine. Check with your state medical board or other appropriate licensing agency to find out what requirements have been established in your state.

Homeopathy

The principles of homeopathic medicine are popular around the world today. This type of whole medical system views illness as a disturbance in a person's vital force. A fundamental law states that a substance that causes certain symptoms in healthy people can be used to treat similar symptoms in people who are ill. Symptoms are signs that your body is trying to heal itself. So by eliciting specific illness symptoms, the remedies are thought to stimulate your immune system and speed recuperation from infirmity and disease.

Homeopathic medicines are composed of animal, mineral, plant or chemical substances. The substances can be used singly or in combination, and in low or high dilutions. Some remedies are so dilute that they contain no residual molecules of the original medicinal substance. In this situation, all that remains is the energy or essence of the original substance which, purportedly, becomes transferred to the dispensing vehicle. According to homeopathic belief, these highly dilute medicines are the strongest and most potent for treating illness.

Two main types of homeopathy exist. The first one is constitutional, or classical, homeopathy. The other kind is disease-oriented or symptomatic homeopathy. As part of the healing process, a temporary worsening of your symptoms can sometimes occur initially using either method.

Constitutional Homeopathy

This branch of homeopathy views physical symptoms as more superficial than ones that are mental or emotional. It aims to find and treat the underlying causes of deeply buried disorders and chronic diseases. It does this by looking at the complete symptom picture of an individual.

A practitioner of constitutional, or classical, homeopathy analyzes physical, mental, emotional, hereditary and lifestyle data from a patient to choose an appropriate remedy. A treatment is chosen that closely matches the patient's individual details. Very dilute remedies that are reputed to have higher potencies are usually prescribed after a complete and thorough evaluation.

Disease-Oriented Homeopathy

Medicines are given for specific, symptomatic health conditions in this form of homeopathy. The remedies are available over-the-counter for consumers who purchase them for self-care. Typically, the medicines are prepared at low dilutions, which are seen as milder, and often contain a combination of ingredients.

Homeopathic remedies are regulated the same as over-the-counter drugs by the U.S. Food and Drug Administration. Due to regulation differences, you may notice that homeopathic medicines are allowed to make healing claims on their labels, while herbs and dietary supplements are not.

The following are examples of homeopathic remedies commonly in use for allergies.

Allium cepa

Derived from onion, this homeopathic remedy is used to treat people who have problems with profusely watery eyes or a nose that runs continuously. The remedy is commonly used for allergic rhinitis, eye allergies, colds and runny noses.

Galphimia glauca

Some evidence indicates that homeopathic preparations of *Galphimia glauca* may be helpful for the eye symptoms of hay fever such as itchy or watery eyes. It may also be helpful if the symptom complex includes swollen eyelids, sneezing, skin rash, and sensitivity to weather change.

Euphorbium

Euphorbium is a mixture of juices from several different species of euphorbia plants. A homeopathic treatment containing euphorbium may alleviate allergic sinus problems. Nasal congestion and sinus pressure showed significant improvement in one study. Euphorbium may also provide benefit if the symptom complex includes a watery nasal discharge, frequent sneezing, headache, dizziness and difficulty breathing.

Eyebright (Euphrasia)

Eye allergies are sometimes treated with eyebright. It is traditionally used as a poultice, eyewash, or eyebath. The effectiveness of eyebright is questionable based on research. *Caution*: Since medicine placed in the eye can cause irritation or infection, use eyebright only under the supervision of a physician.

Isopathic remedies

These medicines represent a special case. Standard homeopathic remedies are made from a variety of substances that produce the symptoms of illness in healthy people; the remedies are then used to treat similar symptoms in people who are ill. But isopathic remedies are prepared from the precise substance that triggers the patient's disorder. For example, a patient with cat allergies might be given a dilute homeopathic mixture derived from cat hair. Several studies show beneficial results after the treatment of allergic individuals with isopathic remedies. *Caution*: The remedies should be used only under a qualified physician's supervision.

Part IV
Prevention of Allergic Conditions

৪৩৫৪৩

Chapter 15
Allergy Prevention

☙❧

What a wonderful thing it would be to prevent allergies from occurring in the first place. How could we do that? Scientists in the field have discovered several possibilities. Let's look at what's known about modifying risk factors for allergy prevention, starting at the beginning.

In early infancy a critical period exists during which time susceptible children may begin to develop allergies. Research indicates that environmental factors play a role as do contact with allergens and a child's family history. Having a parent or sibling with an allergic condition such as hay fever, asthma, eczema or food allergies places a child at increased risk for developing a similar disorder. Many studies have looked at high-risk children to determine what changes can be made during their first few years of life to lower allergy risk.

Diet & Lifestyle Changes

Based on the evidence to date, pediatric experts often provide the following advice about how to prevent allergies in children:

- Breastfeed your child for at least six months. Human milk is the best source of nutrition for full-term infants.
- Supplement or wean with a hypoallergenic formula that is extensively hydrolyzed, or pre-digested. Partially hydrolyzed formulas are somewhat more allergenic. Avoid the use of conventional cow's milk formulas and soy formulas since they have not been found to reduce allergies. Talk to your child's doctor for brand recommendations.
- Avoid cow's milk in all infants under the age of one year.
- Introduce solid foods to children at four to six months of age. Previous advice to delay solid foods in children at risk for allergies has not been supported by recent studies.
- When introducing solid foods, try less allergenic foods first such as rice cereal, pureed fruits, vegetables and meats. If less allergenic foods are tolerated, gradually and carefully introduce more allergenic foods. Contact the child's health care provider if an allergic reaction develops at any point.
- Don't smoke around your child before or after birth.
- May sure your child participates in physical activities nearly every day of the week.
- Encourage consumption of fruits and vegetables and limit processed foods and soft drinks.

Keep in mind that there is still considerable debate about the safety and effectiveness of specific measures for allergy prevention. Always consult with your child's health care provider before making dietary or lifestyle changes that would affect your child, especially when there is a history of severe allergies.

Elizabeth Smoots MD

Friendly Intestinal Flora

A fascinating area of prevention research involves the friendly bacteria in your gut. Mounting evidence suggests these bacteria play an important role in allergy formation and prevention. Beneficial bacteria in adequate amounts help regulate and guide normal maturation of your immune system. They also act in ways that decrease inflammation and subsequent damage to the lining of your gut. Conversely, a shortfall in the diversity or quantity of gut bacteria early in life may predispose people to the later development of allergies.

One line of evidence shows that children born by cesarean section may have an increased risk of asthma and allergies. Babies normally receive a small amount of their mother's intestinal flora during vaginal delivery. But infants born by cesarean section miss that opportunity. Instead, the c-section babies acquire disturbances in their gut microbial composition. Studies show the babies have fewer beneficial bacteria such as *Lactobacillus*, and more potentially harmful ones like *Staphylococcus* and *Acinetobacter*. The bacterial imbalance can predispose them to allergic disease, according to accumulating evidence.

Other research indicates that children who repeatedly receive broad-spectrum antibiotics during early life are prone to developing allergic conditions like asthma. The antibiotics kill off friendly bacteria and allow unfriendly ones to grow. Imbalances in the children's gut bacteria may set the stage for subsequent allergies.

Based on this evidence, we could in theory modify risk by giving beneficial bacteria in the form of probiotics and prebiotics to allergy-prone individuals. Probiotics are live microorganisms that are consumed for their health benefits. The most common sources of probiotics are foods such as yogurt, buttermilk, kefir, raw sauerkraut, and other cultured or fermented foods.

Prebiotics are indigestible food ingredients that can stimulate the growth of beneficial bacteria in the colon. Typically, prebiotics come from foods rich in soluble fiber like fruit, leafy greens, onions, beans, flaxseeds, oatmeal, barley and other whole grains. Early research on the use of probiotics and prebiotics for the prevention of allergies has shown promise, but further studies are needed.

In the meantime, be aware that even beneficial bacteria may potentially have adverse effects. Check with your health care provider before giving probiotics or prebiotics to susceptible groups of people. At the top of the list of groups are infants, the elderly, and those with chronic disorders or weak immune systems.

Future research will likely identify additional promising areas as the search continues for effective methods of allergy prevention.

Elizabeth Smoots MD

Appendices
୬୦ଔ

Appendix A
Sample Elimination Diet

CR80

Here I've shown a sample elimination diet with examples of foods that are commonly allowed or avoided in the main food categories. You can modify the plan's general framework to fit your needs. For example, if you notice a particular allergy or sensitivity, add that food to your list of foods to avoid during the elimination phase of your diet. Be sure to eat regular meals and snacks to maintain your energy level, and drink plenty of fluids to avoid dehydration.

Animal Protein
Allowed foods: Fresh or water-packed canned chicken, turkey, duck, lamb, wild game, cold-water fish
Foods to avoid: Beef, veal, pork, processed meat such as sausage and cold cuts, shellfish, eggs, egg substitutes

Dairy Products
Allowed foods: Rice milk
Foods to avoid: Milk and dairy products from cows and goats, including cheese, cottage cheese, yogurt, butter, sour cream, cream, ice cream; non-dairy creamers

Legumes
Allowed foods: All dried beans except for soybeans, dried peas, lentils
Foods to avoid: Soy products, including soy sauce, soybean oil, tempeh, tofu, soy milk, soy yogurt, textured vegetable protein

Vegetables

Allowed foods: All raw, steamed, sautéed, juiced or roasted vegetables

Foods to avoid: Corn, creamed vegetables

Note: If you have arthritis or joint problems, avoid vegetables in the nightshade family (tomatoes, potatoes, eggplants, peppers, paprika, salsa, chili peppers, cayenne, chili powder)

Fruits

Allowed foods: Fresh fruit, unsweetened canned fruit, unsweetened juice

Foods to avoid: Citrus and strawberries

Grains and Starches

Allowed foods: Rice, millet, quinoa, amaranth, buckwheat, teff, potatoes, potato flour, tapioca, arrowroot. This includes breads and cereals made from these foods, and that are free of the ingredients you are trying to eliminate.

Foods to avoid: Products containing corn or gluten. Grains that contain gluten include wheat, barley, spelt, kamut, rye, triticale and malt. Also exclude oats since they are often contaminated with gluten.

Soups

Allowed foods: Vegetable-based soups without thickening agents

Foods to avoid: Canned or creamed soups

Beverages

Allowed foods: Unsweetened fruit and vegetable juices, caffeine-free herbal teas, filtered or pure water

Foods to avoid: Dairy, alcohol, citrus drinks, sodas, coffee, tea, caffeinated beverages

Note: If you are used to drinking caffeinated beverages on a regular basis, slowly reduce them before totally eliminating them, to avoid caffeine-withdrawal headaches. To keep energy levels up, eat regular balanced meals and snacks containing protein throughout the day.

Fats

Allowed foods: Cold-pressed or expeller pressed oils made from olive, canola, flax

Foods to avoid: Butter, margarine, shortening, processed oils, nut oils, sesame oil, sunflower oil, pumpkin oil, salad dressings, mayonnaise, spreads

Nuts and Seeds

Allowed foods: Coconut, pine nuts, flax seeds

Foods to avoid: Peanuts, peanut butter, nuts, nut butter, sesame seeds, sunflower seeds, pumpkin seeds

Sweeteners

Allowed foods: Fruit sweeteners, brown rice syrup, agave nectar, stevia, blackstrap molasses

Foods to avoid: White sugar, brown sugar, honey, maple syrup, fructose, sorbitol, molasses, corn syrup, high fructose corn syrup, evaporated cane juice

Chocolate

Allowed foods: None

Foods to avoid: All foods containing chocolate

Processed Foods

Allowed foods: None

Foods to avoid: All processed foods, candy, sweets, chewing gum and other foods with sorbitol

Condiments

Allowed foods: Salt, spices and vinegar

Foods to avoid: Ketchup, mustard, relish, chutney, soy sauce, barbecue sauce, teriyaki and other condiments, including all commercially prepared condiments

Food Additives

Allowed foods: None

Foods to avoid: Foods with artificial colors or flavors, preservatives such as sulfites or nitrites, and other food additives

Elizabeth Smoots MD

Appendix B
Moved to Exercise
The key is getting and staying motivated

ᘓᘓᘓ

If you have trouble sticking with exercise, you are not alone. An estimated 80 percent of Americans don't get enough exercise, and 60 percent of those who start exercising quit within six months. When it comes to staying with an exercise program, it's important to build habits that will last a lifetime. Here are some tips for the long haul:

- **Find something fun**. Some popular options include dance-exercise, basketball or going for a walk in the beautiful outdoors. Fitness and fun go together, so the better time you're having the greater your chances of sticking with it.

- **Variety is the spice of life**—and exercise. There's no need for boredom when you're busy exploring all the possibilities. For example, alternate an impact activity (jogging, aerobics or tennis) with a light-impact sport (weight lifting or biking) or a non-impact activity (swimming). You'll strengthen different muscle groups and reduce your risk of injury, too.

- **Learn what exercise can do for you.** For some it's feeling physically and mentally better. Others find they have more energy when they exercise regularly. And exercise can often be a great stress releaser as well.

- **Focus on your success**—no matter how small. Many small steps add up to big long-term gains. Don't let one slip or miss stop you; as soon as possible exercise again.

- **Additional motivators** can help keep you on track. You may enjoy listening to audio recordings of music or books on a personal stereo, but do it in a safe place. Try a magazine rack on your stationary bicycle, or exercise while you watch the evening news on TV.

- **Exercise with others**. Joining an exercise group or fitness club can be a great way to work out in a supportive environment. Or exercise with an encouraging friend. And never give up on your efforts—keep exercising!

Why warm up before exercise?

It's often tempting to skip the warm up before you workout. But if you do, your body will miss some quality prep time. The benefits of a pre-exercise warm up include:

Prevention of injuries. Engaging in light activity generates heat in your muscles that helps prepare them for more vigorous exercise. Warm muscles perform better: they're stronger, more coordinated and less likely to cramp. Muscle stiffness also decreases and tendons, ligaments and joints become more supple and flexible. Then, if you need to perform a sudden or forceful movement, your system is primed to handle it with less chance of injury.

Protection for your heart. During warm up your blood begins flowing and your heart rate starts to accelerate. The coronary arteries that supply your heart also dilate by degrees, reducing the risk of heart problems with exertion.

To warm up, gradually increase your activities over 5 to 15 minutes. Try walking or jogging in place, stationary cycling, or moves specific to your sport. The sport-specific movements are particularly helpful since they provide dynamic stretching

Elizabeth Smoots MD

for the muscles you are about to use. After your movements have warmed and increased the flexibility of your muscles, you can begin to pick up your exercise pace.

Contrary to popular belief, the best time to work on static flexibility is at the end of your workout after your muscles are completely warmed up. Static stretching elongates your muscles during rest. At the end of every exercise session, go through a four to six minute series of static stretches for your whole body. Each stretch should be done slowly and steadily without bouncing, and should not be painful. Stretch each muscle to a comfortable limit for eight to ten seconds, then relax and repeat a couple of times.

Appendix C
How Much Calcium Are You Getting from Food?

ᏟᎡᏜᎧ

Consuming calcium-rich foods is a great way to make sure you're getting enough calcium and other minerals for good health. You need calcium for your bones as well as for normal muscle contractions, heart rhythm, enzyme functioning and blood clotting. But many men, women and children in the U.S. do not consume adequate amounts of calcium.

Here I've summarized the best sources for getting calcium from food.

Dairy products. Milk, yogurt, cheese and other dairy products are an excellent source of readily absorbed calcium. But people with milk allergy must avoid them, and those with lactose intolerance may want to limit their use.

Other animal sources. Shrimp, oysters and canned fish with the bones such as salmon, sardines, and mackerel are all excellent sources.

Leafy greens. Readily absorbed calcium in plentiful supply is found in members of the cabbage family such as kale, bok choy, broccoli, mustard greens, collards and turnip greens. Other good calcium sources include dandelion greens, parsley and romaine. The calcium in members of the beet family is not as bio-available since it's bound by oxalic acid; members include beet greens, spinach and chard.

Legumes. Beans, lentils, peas and soy products such as soy milk and tofu are sources of calcium.

Other plant foods. Peanuts, nuts, sesame seeds and sunflower seeds contain ample amounts of calcium. Seas vegetables like nori, kombu, wakame and agar-agar are also good sources.

Fortified foods. Products such as orange juice, rice milk, almond milk, cereal, bread and tortillas are sometimes fortified with calcium. Check the label for the amount of calcium per serving.

For a list of the calcium content of foods

See Appendix D.

How much calcium do you need?

The Institute of Medicine recommends the following daily allowances according to gender and age group:

- 9-18 years: 1,300 mg
- 19-50 years: 1,000 mg
- Pregnant or lactating females aged 19-50 years: 1,000 mg
- 51-70 year-old females: 1,200 mg
- 51-70 year-old males: 1,000 mg
- Females and males older than 70 years: 1,200 mg

Estimate your daily calcium intake

Pick a day and record the amounts and types of food that you ate on that day. For each of the calcium-rich foods that you consumed, multiply the number of servings you had by the calcium content of that food. (See Appendix B for the calcium content of select foods.) This will tell you how much calcium you received from that food. Do the same for all of the calcium-rich foods you had on that day and then add them together. The sum is the estimated total amount of calcium you got from all of the food you consumed on that day.

If your calcium intake varies a lot from day to day, check your calcium intake on three or four fairly representative days, and average them together. Compare your average daily calcium intake to the recommended daily allowance of calcium for your age and gender. If your intake is lower than recommended, you can eat more calcium-rich food or talk to your physician about taking a supplement.

Appendix D
Calcium Content of Select Calcium-Rich Foods

❧

Calcium content can vary markedly between different food samples and products. Check the label or product information of each product you are using for specific calcium amounts. Here is the calcium content of selected calcium-rich foods as recorded by the United States Department of Agriculture.

Beans, black, cooked, 46 mg in 1 cup
Beans, great northern, cooked, 120 mg in 1 cup
Beans, kidney, cooked, 50 mg in 1 cup
Beans, navy, cooked, 126 mg in 1 cup
Beans, pinto, cooked, 79 mg in 1 cup
Cereal, calcium-fortified, 100 mg in 1 cup
Cheese, 204 mg in 1 oz
Cheese, cottage, 138 mg in 1 cup
Greens, bok choy, cooked, 158 mg in 1 cup
Greens, broccoli, cooked, 62 mg in 1 cup
Greens, collard, cooked, 268 mg in 1 cup
Greens, kale, cooked, 94 mg in 1 cup
Greens, mustard, cooked, 165 mg in 1 cup
Greens, parsley, raw, 83 mg in 1 cup
Greens, romaine, raw, 16 mg in 1 cup
Greens, spinach, cooked, 245 mg in 1 cup
Greens, spinach, raw, 30 mg in 1 cup
Greens, turnip, cooked, 197 mg in 1 cup
Lentils, cooked, 38 mg in 1 cup

Milk, cow's, nonfat, 299 mg in 1 cup

Milk, cow's, 1% fat, 305 mg in 1 cup

Milk, cow's 2% fat, 293 mg in 1 cup

Milk, cow's, whole, 276 mg in 1 cup

Milk, goat's, 327 mg in 1 cup

Milk, rice, 283 mg in 1 cup

Milk, soy, 299 mg in 1 cup

Nuts, almonds, 75 mg in 1 oz

Nuts, hazelnuts, 32 mg in 1 oz

Nuts, pecans, 20 mg in 1 oz

Nuts, walnuts, 28 mg in 1 oz

Orange juice, fortified, 349 mg in 1 cup

Peas, split, dry, cooked, 27 mg in 1 cup

Salmon, cooked with bones, 273 mg in 4 oz

Sardines, cooked with bones, 274 mg in 4 oz

Seaweed, agar, dried, 179 mg in 1 oz

Seeds, sesame, whole, 279 mg in 1 oz

Seeds, sesame, hull removed, 17 mg in 1 oz

Seeds, sunflower, hull removed, 22 mg in 1 oz

Shrimp, cooked, 104 mg in 4 oz

Shrimp, canned, 166 mg in 4 oz

Tofu, firm, 206 mg in 4 oz

Yogurt, plain, low fat, 448 in 1 cup

Yogurt, plain, nonfat, 488 mg in 1 cup

Source: National Nutrient Database for Standard Reference, United States Department of Agriculture

Elizabeth Smoots MD

Appendix E
The "Dirty Dozen"

ᘓ᠘ᐱ

Organic foods have significant health benefits but can be costly. If you are on a budget, consider buying organic versions of the fruits and vegetables that are most heavily treated with pesticides. Going organic for these 12 foods can reduce your pesticide exposure by as much as 90 percent, according to tests done by the Environmental Working Group, a nonprofit research organization based in Washington, D.C. The list places the fruits and vegetables with the highest pesticide loads at the top.

1. Apples
2. Celery
3. Sweet bell peppers
4. Peaches
5. Strawberries
6. Nectarines (imported)
7. Grapes
8. Spinach
9. Lettuce
10. Cucumbers
11. Blueberries (domestic)
12. Potatoes

Additionally, green beans and kale may contain pesticide residues of special concern. For more information, go to *www.ewg.org.*

Appendix F
The "Clean Fifteen"

Œ₹&O

The following fruits and vegetables are likely to be lowest in pesticide contamination, according to tests done by the Environmental Working Group, a nonprofit research organization based in Washington, D.C. If you are on a budget, you may consider eating non-organic versions of them. The list places the fruits and vegetables with the lowest pesticide loads at the top. For more information, go to *www.ewg.com*.

1. Onions
2. Sweet corn
3. Pineapples
4. Avocado
5. Cabbage
6. Sweet peas
7. Asparagus
8. Mangoes
9. Eggplant
10. Kiwi
11. Cantaloupe (domestic)
12. Sweet potatoes
13. Grapefruit
14. Watermelon
15. Mushrooms

Appendix G
Glossary of Herbal & Botanical Terms

ℭℛℰᴏ

Crude bulk herb
An herb that is dried and left intact. Crude bulk herbs can be prepared from almost any part of an herb or plant.

Crude powdered herb
An herb that is dried and then powdered. Crude powdered herbs can be prepared from almost any part of an herb or plant.

Decoction
An herbal preparation, or tea, made by combining an herb with water and bringing the mixture to a boil, then simmering for five to ten minutes. Strain before drinking. Herbal decoctions are usually prepared from sturdy plant parts such as roots or bark.

Extract
A general term for an herbal preparation made by pulling out the active principles of a plant using a solvent such as alcohol or water. The extract contains the plant's essence in concentrated form. Extracts made be prepared as liquids such as tinctures, or they may be made in dry, powdered form.

Glycerite
An herbal preparation made by combining an herb with a mixture of glycerin and water. Glycerites are sometimes used for children or those sensitive to alcohol.

Infusion

An herbal preparation, or tea, made by pouring hot, boiling water over a fresh or dry herb placed in a cup or bowl. Cover the mixture and let sit (steep) for five or ten minutes or more, then strain. Herbal infusions are usually prepared from delicate plant parts such as flowers, leaves or seeds. The infusions are sometimes called "tisanes."

Maceration

An herbal preparation, or tea, made by soaking an herb in cold or room temperature water. Let sit (steep) for six to eight hours at room temperature. Macerations are also called "cold macerations" or "cold infusions."

Standardized extract

An herbal extract that contains a specific amount of an active ingredient or marker compound. The amount of ingredient is quantified and printed on the label.

Tincture

An herbal preparation made by combining an herb with a mixture of alcohol and water. The mixture is steeped at room temperature for a couple of weeks and then strained. Tinctures have much greater potency than teas.

Elizabeth Smoots MD

About the Author

ଔଓ

Sample from Dr. Elizabeth's Blog
A Whole Health Life

CRREO

Join Dr. Elizabeth Smoots as she writes about the whole health life and holistic integrative medicine in her blog *A Whole Health Life: Finding wellness of body, mind and spirit.* She keeps you posted on alternative and conventional approaches that—alone or in combination—can foster wellness of your complete self. Finding balance for your body, mind and spirit is a path you can travel a step at a time.

Following is a sample blog post from *A Whole Health Life.* You can view additional posts at *www.drsmoots.com.*

Living a Whole Health Life

⳩⳪

A whole health life is filled with total health for you. Living such a life encourages holistic health, or wellness of all parts of you, including your mind, body and spirit. The idea of holistic health has been largely forgotten in our modern world. But I think the time is past due to bring the holistic concept back into our lives and our health care system.

It would be silly to think that you are a stomach or an eye or a brain. Yet, this is how conventional medicine thinks of you. You're advised to go to an ophthalmologist, or eye specialist, if something is wrong with your eyes. You're told to see a counselor if you want to talk about your mental health or emotional issues. And you may be asked to visit a gastroenterologist, or stomach expert, to get help for your digestive ills. But really, you are much more than the sum of your parts and are a complete being with a body, mind and spirit that are interwoven and inseparable.

An emerging field called integrative medicine looks at people comprehensively and holistically. It does this by combining principles from both alternative and conventional care. Preventive therapies like diet, exercise and healthy lifestyle habits form the foundation of integrative medicine. Practitioners emphasize building a partnership with patients to provide better care for the mind, body and spirit.

The specialty of integrative medicine embraces evidence-based alternative approaches to treating illness. Examples of popular alternatives include herbal remedies, dietary supplements, meditation, breathing exercises, hypnosis, guided imagery, acupuncture, homeopathy, chiropractic or osteopathic manipulation, and massage therapy. Integrative

Elizabeth Smoots MD

medicine also recognizes that conventional therapies such as medications or surgery are the most effective options for treating certain disorders.

A Whole Health Life is aimed at helping people like you live a life filled with whole health. The ultimate goal we may achieve is to find complete physical, social, spiritual and mental wellbeing—not merely the absence of disease. In this blog I plan to share my thoughts about the emerging field of integrative medicine. I'll write about alternative and conventional approaches that, either alone or in combination, can foster wellness of your complete self. Come along on the journey as we explore what it means to lead a whole health life.

Excerpted from Dr. Smoots' Blog
A Whole Health Life
www.drsmoots.com

Biography
Dr. Elizabeth Smoots

⳥⳦

Elizabeth S. Smoots, MD, FAAFP, ABFM, is a board-certified family physician with many years of experience in family medicine and primary care. She has long cared for patients in private practice as well as in several group-practice clinics in the Seattle area. In addition to providing primary care for her patients, Dr. Smoots has special interests in women's health, skin conditions, sports medicine, fitness and nutrition as well as preventative and alternative approaches to optimizing health.

A keen interest in integrative medicine led to her completion of a two-year fellowship at the world-renowned Arizona Center for Integrative Medicine, founded by Andrew Weil, MD, at the University of Arizona. As an integrative physician, Dr. Smoots embraces therapies from both the conventional and alternative medical fields and enjoys collaborating with patients to find the right treatment mix for them. She strives to address the mind, body and spirit of her patients and makes use of all appropriate therapeutic approaches to help them achieve optimum health.

Dr. Smoots also has a longstanding personal interest in preventive medicine and patient education. She especially enjoys educating her patients about the prevention and treatment of their medical disorders and health conditions. Her wellness articles have appeared in numerous magazines, newspapers, newsletters and websites, including the *Harvard Health Letter, Personal Best Healthlines, TopHealth, Family*

Safety & Health, Medscape.com, Healthgate.com and WebMD.com. She has long written the syndicated health column *Practical Prevention* for newspapers in the U.S. Additionally, Dr. Smoots has designed an engaging and motivating prevention education program that other physicians can use to educate their patients about staying healthy, fit and well.

Dr. Smoots' credentials include an M.D. from University of Arizona College of Medicine and a B.S. in Biology from Arizona State University. She completed a residency in family medicine at Good Samaritan Hospital in Phoenix, Arizona. Board-certified by the American Board of Family Medicine, she has also been awarded the title of Fellow of the American Academy of Family Physicians. In addition, Dr. Smoots has been honored with a recognition award for long-term service and contributions to the American Academy of Family Physicians.

Dr. Smoots' website contains a wealth of information. In addition to reading her blog, *A Whole Health Life*, you can find out about upcoming additions to the Smoots Guides series. Each book in the series presents integrative solutions to common health problems. The site also provides information about Dr. Smoots' *Practical Prevention* newspaper column and patient prevention education program by the same name. For more information, go to *www.drsmoots.com.*

Made in the USA
Charleston, SC
03 October 2013